I'm Still Standing
Life's for Living

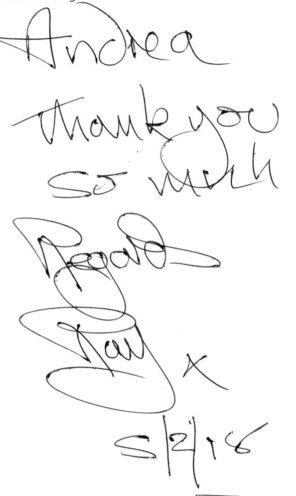

Andrea

thank you
so much.

Regards

Paul x

5/2/16

This book is dedicated to my children:

Diana, Michael, Chris, Nicola and Taya.

I'm Still Standing

Life's for Living

Ray Edwards MBE

with Sally Cope

I'm Still Standing
Life's for Living

First published in 2014 by

Panoma Press Ltd
48 St Vincent Drive, St Albans, Herts, AL1 5SJ, UK
info@panomapress.com
www.panomapress.com

Book layout by Michael Inns
Artwork by Karen Gladwell

ISBN 978-1-909623-70-5

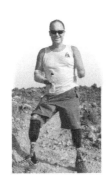

Contents

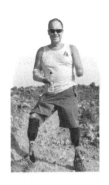

Foreword
Ray, the inspirer!

When you meet Ray, the first thing that greets you is his big smile and his warm welcome. This is what I was faced with when I first met him in April 2013. I was attending visitors' day at a local breakfast business meeting. I was there to promote my property business. Ray was there, with Dennis Outridge, to promote Limbcare. The meeting began at 6.30am, so at that time in the morning it is difficult to be cheerful and chatty, yet Ray managed it, despite having been up since 5am, as he later revealed.

During the meeting we stand up and talk about our business for 60 seconds. When Ray stood up he spoke not for 60 seconds, but for 600 seconds – ten minutes instead of one! No one objected as his talk was inspiring. By the time he answered our questions about his life and Limbcare, the format of the meeting had completely gone. We were all awestruck. Ray had put his mark on the meeting, as he does everywhere he goes. Someone said he should write a book. His quick reply was, "I can't write!" holding up his ilimb. Typical Ray, joking about his disability.

I was so inspired by him I told him I would write his book. He told me to email him. I thought he must get so many people offering I would not hear from him again, especially as I had no experience in writing a book. How wrong could I be!

Ray replied to my email and we booked a time to meet. We hit it off straight away. There were so many things I could relate to: where he lived; Roehampton Hospital (opposite where I was brought up) and where he lives now; and his sense of humour! The rest, as they say, is history. We have met on a regular basis since, in a room in the building where Limbcare is based. We often laughed about what the receptionists must have thought when, on a regular basis, Ray asked for a room for us to go into for about an hour, that we were not to be disturbed and when the room was changed, complaining that we were not sure it would work in a different room! (We had got to feel quite at home in the same room every time.)

I have got to know so many people connected with Limbcare, including Dennis, Barry and John, mentioned in this book. I have been to Ray's house, met his family, including Fiona who is as lovely as he portrays and had a superb time at the Gala Dinner in September. Limbcare is now part of my life too. I am now the author of the Prickle stories, part of Limbcare Youth and Izzy Prickle, the editor of the blog page.

I have made such a good friend in Ray and with everyone else at Limbcare. I hope you enjoy reading this book as much as I have enjoyed writing it.

Sally Cope

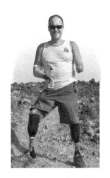

CHAPTER ONE

Young Life

It is good that you don't know what is around the corner. I think if I had a crystal ball to predict the future I would not have known what to do, but I do believe that the basis you have in life helps you through it and I was lucky enough to have a really good, loving childhood to see me through.

Let's start at the beginning. I was born on 5th July 1954, in a nursing home in Hampton Court. The home has now been flattened (I don't know if that is some sort of sign of things to come!). It was by the Cardinal Wolsey pub and my dad went there afterwards to celebrate my birth. Dad was a hard-working man, a builder by trade, and by the time I was born he owned his own company. We lived in Hazelgrove Road, Staines, Middlesex in a fairly typical house for that time, nothing grand. I was the firstborn, so there was plenty of joy and excitement because of my birth. Dad would have been pleased I was a boy, to carry on the family business as was the trend in those days.

Mum told me I was poorly as a baby. My parents were very protective. There were student doctors and nurses around in the hospital and at our local surgery, but Dad wouldn't let them touch me. When I was ill he took me to Dr Sindell, the local GP and his friend, to sort me out with gripe water. I don't know what gripe water does, but it must have worked; my mum seemed to think it did. Dad didn't want anyone else, he only had faith in Dr Sindell, as he knew and trusted him. It seems silly now, as we all have to put our trust in the medical system, whoever is treating us, but I suppose Dad was of the generation where hospitals were for people to die in and to be avoided. How his attitude would have to change in later life!

When I was two or three years old, Dad took over a yard in Egham, Surrey where his company was based and from that moment on, even at such a young age, I was being trained to be a builder. I loved being with my dad and still miss him to this day. He was such a proud dad and so protective of me.

From a young age I always looked up to my dad. He was born in Melton Mowbray, in Leicester, one of four children, the eldest boy. His dad died just after the First World War, due to mustard gas poisoning. My dad was only nine years old, but he took on the role of the man of the family and had to rise to that position very quickly. He must have had a tough time as a child for there was no benefit system and money would have been scarce. This is probably what made him a very strong character. I assume, and I am sure I am right, that this is where I get my strength of character from.

Dad moved down south from Leicester, and met my mum at a dance in Slough. Mum came from a background where her mother and father worked very hard. Just after meeting my mum, Dad decided he wanted to start a building company, so he set one up and it went from strength to strength, but they did work very hard. Both of my parents were very determined people and did everything they could to ensure the family had a good upbringing. Mum always supported Dad, she was a very good wife and mother. My character has been built from Mum and Dad's strength.

I remember being in the yard one day when I was only about three years old. I was watching and copying my dad who was hard at work. A stray dog found its way into the yard. I don't know where it came from and don't remember seeing it, but my dad did, even though he was engrossed with his work. He turned round so quickly, and kicked the dog up the arse in a flash, preventing it from biting me. So protective!

Dad was always very busy. He was out all day getting more work and meeting people to keep the company going, so I never really saw him much until weekends. Dad would always have Saturday afternoon and Sunday off. I loved to help him in the garden, even from a young age. I used to sit in his wheelbarrow while he did the garden. I loved to watch him mowing the lawn, weeding, sitting with him, and building something, watching him. I always liked to help. My initiation into the building trade was, at a very young age, lifting a trowel and helping lay bricks and I loved it.

Dad never shied from hard work and he always liked to be busy. He decided to build a house for the family, so Mum and I stayed in Staines while Dad built the house for us in Englefield Green. One of the things I liked to do most was watch him at work. He had such determination which he passed on to me, thank goodness.

I've talked about Dad, but every engine needs a battery and every man needs a lady behind him. The lady behind my dad was my mum. She was the force who kept everything together: great housewife, great mum. I love my mum. She was such a family person. Even now, I phone her once a week and I see her and she has been such a great friend. I can talk to her about anything. I love her.

When it was time for me to go to school, Mum and Dad decided to send me to a Church of England school; I don't know why, we were not particularly religious. I suppose they thought I would get a good education there. We lived in Englefield Green by the time I was old enough to go to school, so I was sent to St Jude's School. I remember it was a very, very old-fashioned school. I went to school on the back of Mum's bike because she couldn't drive then. It must have looked so funny, but at least I did not have to walk. Everyone used bikes in those days, so maybe it was not as comical as it would be now. Mum did learn to drive eventually, much later. I left that school when I was 11 years old. They built a new one, down the Bagshot Road end of Englefield Green, soon after I left.

Swimming is one of my favourite activities and I still swim every day to keep myself fit, so learning to swim while at school was super. One of my favourite lessons! I still remember the swimming teacher's name and no wonder, as her name was Miss Salmon; I suppose she swam like a fish. Didn't we all laugh! It still makes me laugh today.

I went to Sunday school, every Sunday. Mum would take me and then sit at the back of the church. I enjoyed learning about Jesus and God and loved Sunday school, which is strange, because I am not religious at all.

I never was any good at school; I would rather be helping Dad. I have always been a people person, always liked to talk and do things rather than the academic side of life. I think the talking and communication side has helped me through my later life.

Routine was important in those days, especially at mealtimes. We always ate together, so I would have to wait for Dad to finish work before we had our evening meal. You could always tell what day it was by the food on the table. Sunday was roast, Monday was cold meat, Tuesday was pie, Wednesday chops, Thursday mince, Friday fish and chips and Saturday was pie again. You could run the week, clockwork, by food. There were no big supermarkets, just grocers, butchers etc. I thought it was great and I loved going shopping with my mum. Everyone knew each other, the shopkeepers got to know you by name and they also knew exactly what you wanted on each day. The women shopped every day, as although we had fridges then, they were not used to using them like we are today and old habits die hard. We did not have freezers in our homes; much was fresh produce, so shopping was an important part of the day. I think it was also a way to see each other, to socialise: the men went to the pub, the women went shopping – nothing much changes in that way.

Life changed slightly for the Edwards family when I was eight, as my brother Derek was born. Suddenly with Derek there I thought maybe I was not the 'King Pin' any more. I was not 'The Boy'. I know Mum lost a baby in between me and Derek, so they obviously wanted another baby and it is nice they had what they wanted. I was proud of my baby brother and I remember cuddling Derek when he was a young baby. One time I picked him up and dropped him on the fire hearth; I didn't mean to do it, but that was the way it was. I don't think I realised how much he could wriggle. Luckily I didn't hurt him, but it was always joked that I must have made him a bit weird! The age difference meant that although we got on well, I didn't have much to do with him until we were older. I looked out for him at times. The attention grew away from me a bit, but I was always with Dad until Derek got to an age when I was older, so more independent, living my own life and Dad took on with Derek. It was at this time that Dad formed Edwards Construction Company. Life was good. It was all planned out.

I have had peaks and lows in my life. The start of these lows was so funny really. I was about eight or nine. I came home from school, so excited to tell Mum something. I ran upstairs to find her, couldn't, and so ran straight downstairs without looking, ran into the table, fell over it on to the floor and while I was falling I bit my tongue. Most people would have panicked and rushed me to the local hospital A & E department, but not Dad. As Dad was good friends with the local doctor, as mentioned before, Dr Sindell who worked in Staines, there was no going to A & E (Dad wouldn't have gone there anyway!).

Dad just took me to the doctor's house, knocked on the door, and said, "My son has hurt himself." There was blood everywhere and the doctor just sewed me up. Nowadays that would never happen. This was probably the first time I thought *Oh God, what have I done to myself?*

When I had to leave St Jude's, I didn't get the full achievement there, so I went to Staines Prep School. It was a private school, very different from what I was used to. Looking back, it was quite funny really. They taught me manners: we all had to doff our cap at the head teacher and it was "Good morning Ma'am" – a good teaching ground really. We wore yellow blazers with grey trousers – very smart but very different. I don't know what I would think of wearing a yellow jacket nowadays, but then there was no argument. That is what you had to do, no question. I can remember the swimming lessons there, in what was a very old swimming pool. It was partly in the ground and partly above ground, by about four feet. The chap who took us swimming was a groundsman and he taught swimming by having a pole with a strap on it. You laid your stomach in the strap and he ducked you in and you would just start to swim. Some of the boys didn't get to grips with it, but most of us did. I thought it was great fun, but I am not sure how it was supposed to help you. It must have put some boys off swimming for life!

Mr Burgess, the old deputy headmaster, would usually sit in the common room although sometimes he would come and join us in the dining room and he would always cut his food up with a penknife, something I will always remember. I don't know why or for how long he had done this. No one was brave enough to ask him!

It was a very old-fashioned school, run by him and his wife, but I loved it and you can imagine, you are taught a little bit of Ps and Qs along with elocution lessons but I am afraid I was as thick as anything. When I was asked if I was reading a book, the only book I remembered reading was *Treasure Island*, so I didn't come across as the top of the class, but there were certain things I took away from there, like how to dress smart and I have always been smart, all my life. Even since first school, I came home very smart at the end of the day, yet my brother, when he came home, looked like he had been dragged through a hedge backwards.

I was transferred from there, by Mum and Dad, to Magna Carta School in Staines. My God, what a difference!

From the age of 13 going to a school that had everyone from the surrounding estates was so different from what I was used to. I don't mean common, I mean people from all walks of life. When I got to the gates I didn't know anyone there and I was talking posh. They thought *We will have to get this out of him, this is ridiculous*. There is always an initiation ceremony at a school like this. I can picture the wire baskets, the waste baskets in the playground, and to get their own back they would stick you in the waste basket, so your bottom was in there and you couldn't get out. When the bell rang you just sat there, waiting for someone to get you out – that's just one of the tricks. I suppose really you just became a friend of the gang, so you were accepted. You couldn't keep saying "Morning Ma'am" as they would all laugh. That was a learning curve to find out what real life was all about. I had to learn fast. This gave me good standing for years to come: how to accept what you are and adapt according to the environment. It is interesting how in later life you draw on all these experiences at times.

We went on holiday a lot. This was a sign that Dad's business was doing well, because ordinary people didn't go abroad. We went to Malta, on the *QE2*, *The Canberra* – fantastic holidays. I think you don't appreciate things until you look back. How good life was! The upbringing I had has helped me become who I am today. After all, you never know what is round the corner.

I loved riding my bike and swimming. I liked sport, but preferred doing practical work, making and mending things. My dad was the same. He said, "Don't worry son, I never did much at school." We built cars at school, which I loved; it probably started my love of cars, which again has stayed with me all my life.

Dad and Mum had very old-fashioned values, but they were lovely people. Because Dad lost his dad when he was nine years old, from then on he had been top of the tree. You did not pussyfoot around with him. If you had a cold and did not feel like going to school, you still went. He wouldn't mess about. If you were really naughty, he would discipline you as well. Discipline was inbred in me, and respect. I was always told, "Please and thank you do not cost anything." Mum and Dad taught me respect. Dad was very much a strict man and Mum was Mum.

I miss my dad very much. I know I have many of his traits: not suffering fools is one!

As I grew up, so then girls became the attraction. I even bought a motorbike to impress them. I would do anything! Dad thought I needed a hobby and that a musical instrument would be a good idea. He bought me a trumpet and paid for lessons. I don't need to tell you how I got on, only to say that in the words of my music teacher "more crumpet than trumpet" as there was no blowing, just posing. I thought it would attract the girls, but that did not necessarily work. I tried many things to attract the girls. My mum would say it was showing off and she is probably right. I wanted to be noticed by the girls.

I bought a motorbike then, and at 16 we all went into school with motorbikes and I still have friends from my school days and my motorbike days. I think coming from private schooling to a secondary modern really opened my eyes. I did a lot with Dad at weekends with building. I still had my friends, and girls of course. Once I had the mobility of a motorbike I was up and off!

I can remember particularly when I was in my last year at school Dad got to know the chauffeur of one of the Beatles, John Lennon. He had been a lorry driver before becoming a chauffeur. John Lennon was living in Weybridge at the time and Dad had done some road works there, building car parks and erecting fencing. John wanted some work done, so the chauffeur put Dad in touch with him. I said to Dad that I would love to meet John Lennon. By then he had bought a place called Tittenhurst Park in Ascot.

John asked Dad to build a lake, so he called Dad 'Syd the Lake' (Dad's name was Syd). I was lucky and honoured to meet John, I was 16 and he was my hero. This was 1970, he had left the Beatles and was living with Yoko Ono. That was my introduction to famous people.

Looking back, it was a wonderful childhood. Mum and Dad were so good to my brother and me. You couldn't wish for a better childhood. I was really proud of Dad and that was what was set that I would be: a builder.

I left school at the age of 17 with one 'O' level: wood-work. I knew that would not get me very far. I could hardly be a bank manager or an accountant, but I didn't want that anyway. I just liked doing practical things and I had been taught very well by my father, so I started work with Dad, training to become a builder. I was office-bound at first and although I loved it, I really just wanted to go out with the builders. I wanted to be a builder, and learned from the ground up: roadworks, landscaping, I just learned everything.

We moved to Langham Place in Egham and by then my passion for anything mechanical had begun, so I got my first car, an Austin 10, and learned to drive in the back yard. I wish I still had that car, it would be a classic car by now. I passed my test not long after my 17th birthday; I had left school and had begun an apprenticeship with Dad and now I could drive. How impressive was that to the girls! When I look back, those 17 years went so quickly and they were such good fun. We had a beautiful home and a good family relationship. I looked up to my dad, he was a friend as well as a father. When I was 18 he took me to the local pub to buy me a pint, never mind that I had been going to the pub for quite a while. I didn't let on, although I am sure he knew.

When I was 19 Dad decided to leave Egham and move to Bournemouth. I started an apprenticeship at Poole Harbour yacht club, as an assistant bosun. I loved the charisma and charm of the yachts and the smart dress sense: black trousers, white shirt and epaulettes. I especially liked the big occasions, in particular the opening ceremony when the managing director of

Matchbox Toys came to an award ceremony with celebrities in tow. I loved it! The girls loved the uniform too, but that is another story!

There is a funny story of when I became assistant bosun at the yacht club. I loved being dressed up in beautiful clothes: well-creased trousers, polished shoes, white shirt, epaulettes, hat. I was on call. We had a call to say a 40-foot boat *Princess* was coming in. I had to see it in. It was a beautiful afternoon, sun shining and on the bow of the boat (the front) there was a stunning young lady, smiling at me, wearing a bikini, and her dad was steering the boat in towards me. I was in awe. My lip had dropped, my tongue was hanging out, I was there, looking. I was walking while directing the boat in, trying to look really cool, but unfortunately I was not looking where I was going and walked straight off the pier! There was hysterics coming from on board and all they could see was me in the water and the hat floating away. I swam to the hat and retrieved it. Luckily the radio had landed on the pontoon. I got out and was so embarrassed.

I said, "I think you need to moor here."

They said, "Do you need a towel?"

I got a towel and luckily I had spare clothes. It was very embarrassing, but a nice embarrassment because they invited me on board. That was a good day in my life, it was great to meet the family. At the opening ceremony when the yacht club was opened, Dad and I were guests at the marina. It was brilliant. A famous yachtsman, I think it was the person who sailed *Gipsy Moth IV*, came down.

I get my sense of humour from my dad. Things that I found hard I just laughed at.

I did everything at the yacht club: cleaned the toilets, gardening etc. then they found I had a bit of business acumen and so that's what I did and I loved every minute of it.

Dad commuted between Egham and Bournemouth and I was getting restless too. I decided I needed to do something additional, so I did a management course in Bournemouth. Dad was becoming bored with the bungalow in Poole; he wanted to do something else so he had a chance of buying a farm in Elstead in Surrey, which he did. I wasn't into farming at that time and wanted to go back into building, so that is what I did. I went back to Egham to run the building firm, but I enjoyed the contrast between the life of a builder and then on the farm. It was an added bonus of the countryside. It was during this time I learned about employing people: what sort of person you had to be to be successful.

Although I lived in Egham, I helped Dad build the farmhouse and with the animals; we had Suffolk ewes and Red Sussex cattle. He was busy in Egham once and it was March: lambing season. It was left to me and Mum to become the shepherds. Having never been a shepherd it was very difficult, but you certainly knew when the ewes were giving birth to their lambs and sometimes I had to do what they do on *All Creatures Great and Small*: find the head and pull the lamb out. I even had to pull triplets out and I managed it. It is quite an amazing feeling of bringing life into the world, I shall never forget it. We sat there in the top field, in the barn, looking after them and it felt good. I didn't really know what to do, I just followed my instincts.

Unfortunately, come the summer season when it was haymaking time, I found out I suffered with hay fever. I never realised you could suffer so much. Haymaking and hay fever do not go well together. I tried everything I could think of but it was no use, and in the end I wore a mask for protection. I looked like an alien driving a tractor with mask and protector clothes on to prevent the hay fever. It didn't help that much, I was still sneezing in the mask!

The life I enjoyed the most was back in Egham, working on the roads and buildings. It was a great life doing tarmacking, working on the roads and then taking time out to work on the farm. I didn't realise how good life was, but then you don't at the time, you take everything for granted. I never thought in years to come things would happen to change my life completely.

Being the boss's son, the employees were always looking at me, saying, "Oh yeah, he has got a cushy number."

I suppose they see it that I did. I had a car, quite a nice car, money, freedom. In any walk of life you have to prove your position to get respect and to gain respect you have to give respect, but you have to work hard. So my decision was that I didn't want to be an office wallah, I wanted to learn and be part of the team. So I said to Dad that I wanted to be picked up early in the morning by one of the foremen and learn from the ground up. And that is what I did and I did gain respect. It was tough. They used to go in the café in the morning and have their banter, and as the boss's son they thought I was a spy! It took about three months for them to see that I was a worker, gradually going up through the ranks to become a foreman and have my own gang, which is what I did. I think that is where you can gain a lot of knowledge and understand business. You still need to know how to run a business, how the accounts work etc., but if you know your job, you are then OK to go on site and tell people they are not doing it right and how to do it properly. You gain more respect then. This is what I did and I am glad I did it.

I thought life was it: I had a fast car, a Triumph Stag, going out, enjoying myself. I was a bit of a lad with the young ladies and I did get myself a bit of a name. I did like a pint as well. My dad always said that he wanted to buy me a seat in the Kings Arms or the Bells of Ousley, because that is where I normally ended up. I tended to drink a lot as a young man, I suppose that is a trait of a builder, but I did work hard. It was one night in Windsor where I met the girl who was to become my first wife. It was 1978 and now with a steady girlfriend I had it all! Life could not have been better. Derek was happy too, doing his own thing, being a mechanic, all looked quite fine.

Looking back at my childhood has been about school and wanting to work with Dad; if I had learned more and done a lot more studying, would I be any different? Would I still have wanted to work for my dad? No, I don't think I would have done things differently. I liked doing practical things, Dad taught me everything. Going to college and learning management was a good skill, because you understood how to get the best from people, but my art of communication was definitely taught to me by my father. If you are nice to people they are nice back, and when you employ people the same thing applies.

It was getting to the stage where I wanted to move out from the farm and buy a house. I had been with my girlfriend for a while and so we decided to get married and buy a house together. In 1978 we got married in Staines and found a house in Egham. Getting married was really fantastic. My life was beginning to be complete: my own business, own house and now a married man. The house we bought was very old and needed a lot of work doing on it, so I used to finish the day job and then go home and carry on again, completely stripping the house, rebuilding and refurbishing it to create our first home.

The location was perfect because I did not have to walk very far to the yard where I worked. I lived in the house while we were working on it to get it right while she lived in Old Windsor. I got married at the age of 24 and that was when we started to work on the house. Life was great then, my motto was 'live for today and enjoy my life'; it is a good job you do not have a crystal ball to see into the future. This house was built at the turn of the century and there was a lot of dry rot. There were a lot of things we got away with that you wouldn't do now, because of health and safety. One particular job was to get rid of the dry rot with a spray paint. Nowadays you would wear a mask, but in those days I didn't and I was under the floorboards, in a gap about two foot six under the floor. I was breathing in the fumes and you never know if that is what caused a problem a few years later, we just didn't know. I worked very hard including installing new windows, it was a complete refurbishment. Along with working for Dad's company Edwards Construction, I was burning myself out. You don't get ought for nought. You have to put a lot in to get something out of life. I was determined to make good of my life. I enjoyed it; again, my childhood came back into my mind: the fun, laughing and just enjoying ourselves. Money did not seem a worry, but when you become grown up it is a big worry. It is a worry to live. We had the three-day week, and two increases in VAT. You learn a lot running a business and Dad mostly wanted to run the farm. I had some good teams with me, and my brother was working over Guildford way, with Dad on the farm.

I got the house completed in 1980. In 1981 I felt very poorly one day. I happened to be on holiday with my wife. I was still feeling ill when I came back so my dad made me see the doctor who said, "I think you need to go and have a test." I didn't think any more of it and went happily to have the tests, just thinking they would then be able to sort me out and I could get back to work. How little did I know. The tests gave me a result which would lead to my life completely changing: they revealed I had Hodgkin's disease.

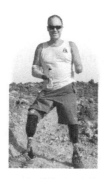

CHAPTER TWO

The S... hits the fan!

So we have just found out that I have been diagnosed with Hodgkin's disease. This was late October/November 1981. When the doctors discover you have a serious illness, you seem to have more tests than you can ever imagine. The tests are bad enough, but the waiting time is the more gruelling at this point. You are in the dark, you don't know what you are about to face and although you try to be positive there is always a nagging doubt in the back of your mind.

You have the tests and then you go to see a consultant. I went to King Edward VII Hospital, Windsor. It is quite frightening when you are told you are seriously ill and need treatment and an operation. For me, the most frightening was the unknown. It was very early days for computers, and we didn't have them at home, so to find out anything you either went to the library or kept asking. I kept asking the consultant about it, I wanted all the details. I wanted to know what the treatment would be. You have a biopsy.

The biopsy was seen to be malignant and we knew they would have to do further tests. Another waiting game…

The first thing that was going to happen was to have internal investigations and my spleen removed. This procedure was done in Princess Margaret Hospital, Windsor by Dr Blaxland, a charming man with a lovely bedside manner. The reason they were removing my spleen was that in those days it was the accepted thing to do if you had Hodgkin's disease. I was happy to go ahead with anything they suggested as I just wanted to get better. I wanted to live and get on with life. I hated being ill and still do. Anyway, what was the problem with removing the spleen? We don't really need it, it is an organ we can live without, but it does mean you have a reduced immune system. My thoughts have now changed: you do need it, because without it you are susceptible to disease and illness. With no spleen your immunity is reduced, so you do need it, but hindsight is a wonderful thing.

I underwent the procedure which involved having a big long cut in my stomach and the spleen removed and the other organs checked out. I was stapled up, lots of staples in my stomach. I went home to recover and by then my blood had been tested and I got the results three weeks later, after recovering from major surgery. This seemed like a long wait, but I was in a positive frame of mind. I wanted to get better and the sooner the better. I am not a good patient, in fact an impatient patient! Just let me get on with things. I know this attitude has been given to me by my dad: no fuss, just get on with it!

I thought I was tough, that I could take anything, but having the staples out was an experience in itself. Believe me, it is hard enough to get staples out of paper, but when you are a human being it is, I think, 100% more painful than taking a staple out of a piece of paper. It's hell! You get hold of anything you can really, including the nurse who is trying to take the staples out. I don't think she expected the reaction I had, me being a big strong builder. I am sure she had heard the words before but you can't help but swear, the words just come out!

After I had had that procedure done, I was feeling a bit better and my stomach was beginning to feel not so sore, I then had the meeting with the consultant. It was just me and my wife in the room with him. We were both so nervous. We did not want to think about what the prognosis would be – after all, I was only 28. We held our breath when he began to talk and I don't think I really heard anything other than the results showed that there was nothing wrong with the internal organs. Thank goodness!

I had X-rays as well and the doctors found that the cancer, the Hodgkin's disease, was in my glands and was affecting the top of my chest, around my neck. What was the next procedure after that? was my question. I wanted to know, was it possible for me to get better? How long would it take? I just wanted to get on with my life.

No one had said this was cancer, they had called it Hodgkin's disease, but I had guessed through research and the questions the doctors were asking. So I said, "This is a form of cancer, isn't it?" and the consultant answered, "Yes."

When I was told that, my wife was crying and you just think about what you have got to tell the family – not a happy picture. They said this was not a high grade of cancer and they could treat it, so the procedure was to have chemotherapy and radiotherapy. The chemo would be done at King Edward VII, Windsor and the radiotherapy was to be done at Hammersmith Hospital. I mention Hammersmith Hospital because later on in this book you will hear more about it, which I didn't realise at the time.

I went home and we reflected on all the information and what had been said; the bombshell was only just beginning to sink in. We shed some tears, and I thought I had better fight it. I am a bit of a fighter and my dad said, "You will be all right." It came into my mind, Dad is OK, he is as strong as an ox and I have to go with his thought.

So the scene was set to have the chemotherapy and the radiotherapy. As soon as I started the chemotherapy it was a gradual deterioration, of my cells really, as the chemotherapy was killing the bad cells. It became obvious that this was going to be horrible: sickness, feeling ill for at least 24 hours after the treatment. Then you can get on with your life for a bit. There was the possibility of losing my hair through the chemotherapy, but luckily I didn't. I am losing it naturally now, but that is another story. I think I asked what else would go on but the shock came when I was told what else could happen.

I did not realise that chemotherapy could kill sperm cells. I couldn't have children, so that brought on another problem for me. What should we do? So I asked the consultant what happens in this situation and she said my best bet was to go to the London Hospital to leave sperm samples before the treatment began because she thought it could kill a lot. So you go through the horrible routine of going to the hospital, and believe me it is old-fashioned ways of going into a cubicle, the semen is put into a little tub, thank you very much, we will put it on record. How impersonal, how humiliating that can be, it was awful! I thought *Not only am I suffering with a form of cancer, now maybe I can never have children*. This was a very difficult concept to get my head around, as I had always assumed I would be a father someday.

There were three to four months of chemotherapy and three months of radiotherapy at Hammersmith, driving up from Egham in Surrey, once a week. The chemotherapy was hard enough, particularly the sickness. The radiotherapy was where you lie on a special bed and you have a lead waistcoat and the opening where they are going to give you the radiation is marked with a blue X on your chest. After a few sessions you are feeling nauseous, but I had become used to that. The worst part was your throat feels as if it has had a hot poker stuck down it and every time you drink, it burns. Even today I still have the hot feeling, causing trouble in the chest area. I was thinking *How long have I got to go through this?*

It continues for as long as it takes, the days turn to weeks, the weeks to months and I had blood tests every few weeks to see how I was doing. Every time I had the tests I wished and prayed the cancer would have cleared. It seemed to go on forever. It had become a way of life, but I didn't want this life. I wanted to get on with things. I wanted my life back, to go back to work, to do all the normal things again. To be young again.

By nine months later, in late summer 1982, I was cleared of the cancer. What a feeling of relief and in many ways disbelief. It felt like I had been ill for ages and now, at last, I could go back to normal, start living my life again, no longer 'ill'. I had to be reassessed every six months, then every year and then every five years, but although there is always a worry in the back of my mind, I am reassured by the check. Thankfully, the cancer has never come back.

But, as I said earlier, the problem was could we have children? Unfortunately, the cancer came when we had just got married and were building our home and life together and now settled in, it would be nice to have children. Well, what do I do? We knew we had the sperm saved at the beginning of the treatment, so do we go to the local hospital to see if

I can get help? Do we want to be childless? For us, that was not really a consideration as we both wanted children. At that time, there was specialised treatment available only at Hammersmith and Wellington Hospital. Hammersmith was via NHS so that was my choice.

We decided to give treatment a go – after all, what had I to lose? I knew I could not have children naturally, so this seemed my only chance. I also wanted to put the cancer behind me and do things normal couples do, and having children was one of those things.

I went to see the Consultant. I had an appointment but I felt like a second-class citizen. I felt was not treated very well and I was not happy with the situation at that time. I had experienced the NHS at first hand and over a long time, but the attitude here was not good. Before the cancer I was a director of the family firm, so I had a good income coming in and we had a little bit saved. I thought *Shall I go the private route?* I felt this was the only route. I attempted to get hold of Professor Ian Craft. It was very difficult to get through, but I was determined, so I waited and waited to see Professor Craft personally and explained the situation.

He said, "Yes, you may come to see us," so we went to see him and started the treatment. It is a totally different ball game when you are a private patient, but remember you are still trying to create a human being by whatever means and unfortunately we had a couple of attempts and that didn't work. This was very difficult to take, not from the cost point of view, which of course was a consideration, but also because it seemed a particularly hard blow since the reason for the treatment was my cancer. So not only had I had cancer, I couldn't become a dad. I was very sad and it caused me a little bit of trauma, quite upsetting really. I wasn't as strong as I thought and we found the childlessness very difficult to deal with. Then her mother died, which was very upsetting, another blow. In all, I was fighting a losing battle.

I went back to work, working for Mum and Dad at their company in Egham, Edwards Construction, and I was working very hard, but I knew things were not right. I was trying hard to please everyone at home and seeing my brother, who had married by now; I was his best man. He started to have children and this caused a bit of anxiety between me and my wife and I found it very difficult. My brother had, by now, become part of the firm; this had happened when I was ill. It made sense for Derek to take my place. I was unable to work when I had the cancer and Dad needed the help, so Derek took my place. But this was hard to accept when I was better, and when Dad told me to come and help my brother I found this very hard. It had always been the other way round, so taking a back seat did not suit me at all.

Dad and all of us were trying to keep the farm going; Dad was on the farm and Derek came to help me, or in reality, I helped him. In my mind, it seemed as if Dad had lost faith in me. This is how I perceived it, although it was not true; he just needed to keep the business going and I had not been able to be around.

I just could not cope with it personally. So to get out of all the pressure I was under, I wanted to start a company on my own. I could only see one way: trying to start my own company, investing all my patience and knowledge to make it work and proving to my dad that maybe I could do something. Although Dad was a hard task-master and cared about both my brother and me, I just wanted to prove who I was. I had to make my own way in life and I missed my friendship with Dad. It wasn't jealousy, because Dad and Derek were similar characters in a lot of ways and I was definitely the worker, out and about doing things. We eventually become great friends. We were a very close family and God, would I give anything to have that back!

I felt I was adding to the family problems because I wasn't giving Mum and Dad any grandchildren. This was the root of the problem. My brother was succeeding: wife, children, running the firm with Dad – and I was failing: no children, and not being around to work for a period of time. I was very unhappy and decided the only way forward was to leave, so I left Dad's company.

I formed Ray Edwards Ltd in 1984. It was a tough decision but I worked hard and it was doing very well. Of course, when you do start on your own you have all the responsibilities of bank loans and worrying about getting work and it is a 24/7 job working for yourself. That created a bit of a rift between me and my family and I became a bit of a black sheep, but I think eventually Dad understood what I was doing.

For the first few years it was tough and we were still trying to have children. When my wife's mum died, I took my wife on holiday and I remember sitting by the swimming pool and saying to her, "I just don't know what to do any more as we can't have children." It seemed this was the only thing I wanted in life – in fact it was what we both longed for.

But I was still trying to prove that I could be successful and that the cancer had not stopped me. So I focused on my business and put children to the back of my mind. I became very successful through determination and sheer bloody-mindedness. I knew what I wanted and went out to get it. I am sure Dad was very proud of me. He could see I had to stand on my own two feet and do things my way. That remains today.

When the brakes come off and you are not trying to have children, miracles happen and with the help of the treatment, giving me quite high doses of drugs to produce whatever there was left, my wife became pregnant. It was the most unbelievable thing. At last we could be a family and I felt I was whole again. I had shown I was a man.

On June 4th 1986 my wife gave birth to twins: a boy and a girl, Michael and Diana. I think the beam on my face then was the biggest ever seen.

With twins though, my God, it is not just one feed, it's two. And given the way I am, it wasn't easy. I was determined to be a good dad and do everything: I was not only providing a roof over our heads for my wife, I was providing for my twins now, my family. But of course, I still had my company to run, to provide a home for the family and so I worked hard and then came home and tried to help out too. For any father of young children it is tiring. Forgive me, I know it is tiring for the mother too, but I am trying to show that keeping all the plates spinning, so to speak, is difficult, but I also had the added pressure of no immune system, so fatigue would at times get the better of me and I would fight it. I was still working very hard, then going home to the twins, but I was a happy bunny. Things were tough and it occurred to me that maybe I was working too hard, but that was life.

I was very tired, and I remember when the twins were christened people said, "You look worn out, Ray." Well, I suppose you would really, and lack of sleep, that is an added thing, but it is just the way it is when you are working hard to become successful. I didn't want people to sympathise with me, I wanted to just get on with life. But their comments began to ring bells in my mind and after June 1986, when the twins were born, I began to think about my responsibilities. The christening comments made me look at insurance for myself, something I had never thought of before. I think I thought I was invincible, but having the twins made me grow up a bit.

I met an insurance broker who said to me, "I think we need to look at insurance," so it was probably January/February time in 1987 that I took out what they call a personal health insurance policy.

One particular question was: "Do you work with trees or dangerous objects?"

I said, "I do roadworks, I do groundworks, I drive JCBs, so yes, I do have to chop down trees sometimes to do landscaping. Why do you ask?"

He replied, "If you lost a limb and were unable to work, you need to take out personal health insurance to help you."

I thought it may be a good idea, as I was a working director. I paid the first month's premium in February that year, to cover any problems. Maybe something was on my side, maybe it was a premonition. Who knows? All I know is it was a good move as things turned out.

I was called out in March to one of the contracts, Fuller Smith & Turner at the Wagon and Horses in Addlestone; we had a call saying that the pub had a problem. We had two gangs working for us then and they were out on contracts already. I did have a mobile phone in those days but it wasn't as neat as they are now. If you can imagine a brick being the battery, the phone, which was Panasonic or Motorola, was heavy and large. The battery didn't last very long, but that was the only kind of mobile phone we had and I had a phone in the car, which looked like a normal phone with a lead. I had a call and I said I would go there. I had a meeting to arrange to visit a client to do an estimate and I called into the pub on the way. I got there first and decided to assess the problem, so I could direct the gang on what to do and this would speed up the process. The problem was there was a blockage which caused a temporary close-down of one of their toilets. Of course for a pub it was bad, because if you can't use the toilet, the pub cannot open. What to do? Should I stay there and sort it? I was suited and booted, ready for my meeting, but I could see the urgency of this problem.

I said to the landlord, "I haven't got any tools, but I need to investigate this quickly." I had a thought to get a camera survey team to investigate where the blockage was. I called them in but they could not get there for half an hour. By then I had taken my shirt off, stripped down to just my suit trousers, ready to see if I could begin to find the blockage. I asked the landlord for a pickaxe and fork. I knew there was a cover somewhere, a manhole cover. I worked out it was somewhere in the area of ground outside his kitchen; underneath the old tarmac must be the manhole. I began digging away, trying to get at the hole, and suddenly I felt a cast-iron cover. You can feel it when you hit it with a pickaxe! I cleared the area and by then the survey team had arrived. They were going to put a camera down the unit to see into the manhole chamber on the screen to identify the particular manhole. We worked out I was in the right area, so I picked up the cover and exposed the opening. The cover was not easy to get up and in doing so I caught my hand on a bit of steel that was sticking out of the cover.

I didn't think much of it, I just wanted to find and solve the problem.

When I opened the cover, the smell from the hole was terrible. I can still remember it to this day. There was something seriously wrong. We had opened up a massive sewer. When the camera was put down we could see what had happened. There was a tree root which had penetrated through the porcelain chamber and blocked the whole thing. By then, the cut on my hand was not looking good. It was open and exposed, but I was more concerned about the manhole problem than my hand. The smell, or rather the stink, was poisonous. I managed to get my team who were working locally to get there and do the job: clear it out and job done. We cleared up, left there and went on our way. I called into a few more sites and went home and thought no more of it, other than dressing my cut. On my way home, I stopped off at The Bird in Hand pub for a drink. How ironic was the name of that pub to be in a very short space of time!

That night I had a splitting headache and I didn't feel well. I thought I was going down with a cold or the flu. By then it was the weekend and whatever I did didn't help. Come Saturday evening/Sunday I was worse: I couldn't move from my bed I felt so ill. I didn't know what was going on. On the Sunday it was my dad's birthday, 1st March and he was coming round for dinner with Mum. I don't know what happened. I could not get out of bed, I only know he came up to me in bed, he picked me up and helped me down the stairs and took me to the Princess

Margaret Hospital in Windsor. I didn't resist. I just wanted to feel better. I could not explain why I felt so bad. The only thing I had done was cut my hand on the Friday. I would find out later that it would seem I had poison in my body, which had gone through my body from, believe it or not, that cut.

I don't remember too much. All I know is that I was in septic shock; my kidneys had started to fail and things were really bad. I remember a Greek doctor who was on call at the Princess Margaret Hospital who probably saved my life, through giving me an intravenous drip. He realised that my kidneys were failing and things were not working right. As I said earlier, having no spleen caused problems. The spleen is told that there is poison in the body and then works on it; with no spleen, the poison can go straight to the heart. The heart reacts, pushing all the poison out and in that case my body was shutting down. I was 'blue lighted': an ambulance with blue flashing lights was called to take me from Princess Margaret to Hammersmith Hospital to go on the renal ward to get emergency treatment.

So this particular part of my life was developing into a trauma. I didn't understand. I really couldn't understand what was going on. I do remember my wife being in the ambulance. I said, "Am I all right?" and then lost consciousness. I didn't know what I could do and that was what I couldn't understand. When we got to the hospital I just remember going through corridors and getting on a bed, but how they did it, I don't know. Everyone was talking about me, not to me, and I really don't remember too much about it. I was in and out of consciousness. Suddenly I was in a bed, I had drips everywhere and I was on kidney dialysis. So, my kidneys had failed. And I know to this day that I did picture two black hands and I heard someone say, "They have got to come off!"

There was a terrible smell around all the time and I could not work out where it was coming from. I am glad I did not know it was my hands. The smell was excruciating.

You can imagine, everyone but me knew it was septicaemia that was the cause and gangrene had set in, so there was dead tissue. I was not in a fit state to know anything. I was in and out of consciousness and all I knew was there was a problem with my kidneys, as I had drips and machines everywhere and people were whispering and talking about me, but not to me. I didn't really care at this time as I was too ill. I just wanted to sleep and wake up feeling better.

What I didn't know was from 1st March they were trying to keep things going, to keep me alive. They were failing. I had septicaemia which was travelling through my body and they needed to act to save my life.

So on Friday 13th March the doctors had to make a big decision. They had to act fast, as things were deteriorating. They rushed me into theatre and amputated not only my hands but my feet too.

This was to save my life.

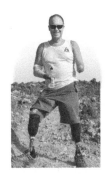

CHAPTER THREE

Teddy Bear

As you can imagine, I didn't really know much about what had happened. The surgeons were removing my arms and legs to save my life. It sounds unbelievable. I'd never heard of this before, but I was in no state to know what was going on. I can't picture the scene in the operating theatre and in some ways I don't want to, because those hours meant my whole life was changing and would never be the same again. There must have been teams of people – one team for each limb. Fancy having to take a person apart like that...

It must have been such an awful decision to make. My parents and my wife had to give their permission for the doctors to operate on me. I never asked them what was said, and again, I don't want to know. It wouldn't change anything. It wouldn't put the clock back. I'm sure it must have been a shock to the doctors and nurses too – all they were trying to do was save my life. I wonder what they were saying to themselves. It's hard to imagine being told that in order to save a life, all the limbs have to be removed.

Eventually the operations were over and I suppose I was in a recovery unit. I don't know how long I was there, I was unconscious and on a lot of drugs. I do remember my father and my wife being there, near to me, sitting with me, but I don't remember what was said.

I remember certain moments of those days, like when I had to be rushed into theatre three more times for operations on one of my legs. There were problems because I was on dialysis which thins the blood, meaning that one of my limbs wouldn't heal. It wouldn't stop bleeding, so they had to try to stem the blood-flow. I can remember one particular night, this was well after 13th March although I don't know exactly when. The doctors said to me, "We just can't stop the blood oozing out of one of the limbs. Can you sign for an operation instead of keep asking your wife to come up?"

I remember them putting a pen next to my stump, which felt terribly wrong. I didn't know about my legs at that point, because I was still sedated. I didn't understand it, but they taped a pen to my right stump and I signed off another operation. It could have been my death warrant for all I knew; I didn't know why I was signing anything, I just wanted to be left in peace.

I don't blame the doctors; they were desperately trying to save my life and take the pressure off my wife. They did their best and succeeded in their mission.

Another day I remember well is my dad having to tell me I'd lost my limbs. He'd been sitting by my bedside, praying for me in his way, pleading with me to please come through. It must have been one of the hardest things he ever had to do. What a thing to have to tell someone, especially your son. He told me about my arms, which I knew because I could see the dressings and I'd 'signed' for the operation with my stump.

It was when he said, "Son, you've got to realise that your legs have been taken off as well."

Well, that was a shock! I had both arms and both legs taken off. I'd known my arms would need to be removed because they were black with gangrene, but the legs were a hell of a shock to the system. Thank God I was on strong drugs because I think I would have sworn the place down, I hadn't realised it was this bad.

I described myself as a teddy bear – I was still on dialysis, so I was even more helpless. That is how I saw myself: useless, unable to do anything. I was totally dependent on everyone else. I lay in the bed, doing the only two things I could manage on my own: looking and thinking. I can remember looking at the floor in the hospital and there were cockroaches scuttling across it. There was an outbreak of cockroaches in this particular hospital and I spent a lot of time just watching cockroaches walk across the floor. I could understand how people who are paralysed feel trapped in their own bodies. I felt trapped too. I felt like a baby, having to have everything done for me. But I wasn't a baby, I was a 32-year-old man.

No arms and no legs at 32. What future had I got? What would I do? I was in a hell hole. In those situations, like soldiers in a war zone, you do think *Oh God, help me.* I wanted it all to be a terrible dream. If it wasn't, I didn't want to live. There was no point living. I wanted to go to sleep and never wake up.

I began to recover slightly and so the nursing staff allowed me to be awake more and even tried to sit me up. It was so degrading to be moved into positions and not be able to move again until they were ready to move me. I wasn't in the best place physically or mentally. People were coming in asking me, "How are we today?"

Well, what a bloody stupid question! How are we? I don't know how they were, but I was p....d off and I didn't like life at all. I didn't know why they'd saved me; I didn't want to be like this, no arms, no legs and on dialysis. What good was I? I couldn't go and build a house. Couldn't walk, couldn't hold things. A living hell.

In and out of consciousness and in my drug-induced state, I remember a visit from a chap I used to know – Ron, the vicar at Englefield Green in Surrey. I don't know why, but to me, whenever a religious person speaks, they speak as if they're singing.

Ron came into the hospital and said, "Oh Ray, how are you?" I don't think I realised who it was, because I told him to fuck off! He went away a bit bemused actually, I don't think he knew what to think or say. Hopefully he realised it was the drugs talking. I would normally never have been so rude to a vicar. My frustration and shock was obviously coming out.

Three weeks later, he came back to see me again. I don't know why, considering how rude I had been to him, but by then my body was coping with getting better and I was in a better place.

I said hello and he said, "Ray, my goodness, it is so nice to see you. You're looking so much better. Last time you told me to go forth and multiply!"

I didn't mean to be horrible and I told Ron I was sorry. He was just pleased to see me. He told me all the people in Englefield Green were praying for me to survive. I didn't want to hear that.

I said, "Ron, look at the state of me – no arms, no legs."

"But you are here."

"But, what can I do?"

Being good friends, he said he was sure I would find a way. He knew I didn't believe in God's way, but sometimes, somehow it will work out. He told me we all go through things for a reason. You must realise that I was listening to so many things that I wasn't sure what to think. I wasn't sure what to believe.

I was a different person. I didn't really feel I was a person. I was someone else. I would have to be rebuilt. Was I up to that? Did I want to face the future and what it would hold for me? The truth is, I didn't know what the future would hold. It was all so alien to me.

When I was in and out of consciousness and able to think a bit more clearly, I heard two people talking about a chapel nearby.

I said to the nurse in charge that day, "Is there any chance of putting me in a wheelchair and throwing me off a cliff?"

She said no. I said, "Second best thing then, take me to the chapel."

I remember this was March and when I looked outside I saw snow. March 1987 was the end of a really bad winter. I wanted to get to the chapel and I wanted to get there now. I'd decided that was the thing to do and nothing was going to stop me, so I slid across the bed. Oh my God... dignity falls out of the window – your arse is sticking out of the bedclothes. It was so frustrating and was making me feel more and more angry and helpless.

There was a wheelchair next to the bed. I couldn't wait for the nurse, I plopped myself into the wheelchair, IV drips everywhere. I remember there were drips in my neck, because the veins were closed off through the arms – well, lack of arms. The nurse came to me quickly, concerned I would fall and hurt myself, but I didn't care. What could I hurt? There was nothing left to hurt! The nurse put me into the wheelchair properly, and then wheeled me to the chapel. I told her to just leave me. I wanted to die and I felt that this would be a good place to go, a peaceful place.

Although it was freezing outside, it was really warm in the chapel. I felt secure from the outside world, like I was in my own cocoon.

But then they closed the door and my God, did it get cold. It was as if a shiver came down my spine. It was really cold, yet the heating was on. Something was happening. I looked up at the altar, at the cross, and just asked, "Why?"

I don't know what happened. I stayed looking at the altar and I must have dropped off to sleep, I suppose. It could have been for seconds or for hours, I don't know. I felt a little bit at ease, more at peace with the world, although I didn't know how or why.

I'd been through cancer, but this was the biggest battle yet. I do feel as if there was an aura around me and I felt something touch my shoulder. I opened my eyes and it didn't feel like a human being. I realised someone was saying it would be all right. I don't know what it was, but I had a kind of vision or felt some kind of presence of someone saying, "We will guard you, you will be OK."

The only thing I know is I felt better mentally. It was at that moment that I felt more at ease with my lot and knew I had to carry on fighting.

Reality kicked in and I remembered that I had no legs, no arms, my kidneys were failing, and there were drips everywhere. But now I knew I didn't want to die yet, which was better than when I entered the chapel.

The nurse came back. She was obviously timing me, not allowing me to wallow too much and for too long. I went back to my bed in the hospital and thanked the nurse very much. I didn't know what I was going to do, but

I knew things would change. Seems funny really: 24 hours later, my kidneys began to work independently again, so at least one part of the body was working better.

One of the hardest things to come to terms with was people talking about me, instead of to me. This happened from day one of the illness. Why didn't they tell me what was going on?

I heard comments like, "What are we going to do with Ray? Where is Ray going to go? He needs to be rehabilitated."

So they were trying to kill the poison, which was going eventually, and they were looking at my rehabilitation. I heard someone shout out Roehampton, Stanmore and Scotland. I didn't want to go anywhere. I wanted to stay where I was, in the place I knew and where they knew me, and just disappear.

There were the visits from people, friends. My wife brought my children in, my twins, who sat on my bed. That was such a mix of emotions: the joy of seeing them, but of course they didn't know what had happened. At the young age of nine months, all they could see was tubes in their daddy and they wanted to pull them out. They were just curious but we had to be a bit careful. It was great to see them and they were my saviours. They were the ones I was fighting for.

But on the other side, it broke my heart to see them. I couldn't do the most basic of things. I couldn't pick them up, couldn't feed them, play with them – I couldn't even cuddle them. I tried to be brave and put a smile on my face but I couldn't. It was so soul destroying. I was this teddy bear, but not even a teddy bear who could cuddle. I cried and cried. It was kind of like they were there, but yet they weren't. They needed their daddy.

So my mission, from then on, was to try to get as well as I could and to look forward to the day when I might be able to cuddle them, feed them, stand and even walk with them. I wanted to be a proper daddy again. But I knew it was a long road to travel.

At last the poison was out of my body. It seemed like a long time, but once I was conscious, every minute seemed like an hour. Time goes slowly when all you have to think about is what you can't do any more. Now it was time to learn how to live my life again. Rehabilitation. Having a new life. Being reborn.

I remember my dad coming to see me and he said he'd brought me a can of beer.

I said, "Oh Dad, how am I going to drink that?"

Up until then I'd been fed through tubes, or fed by a nurse. To drink a can of beer you had to hold it for yourself, drink it like everyone else.

The hospital staff, in their ingenuity, made a cup-holder that I could hold on my stump. They put the cup in the cup-holder and poured the beer into the cup. Believe me, that was like nectar to a bee! As a builder that was my staple drink: bitter and lager after work. It's not that I was an alcoholic, but it was wonderful to have a beer and to have a drink with my dad. It was a blessing. It was beautiful. It was so normal! I had tears in my eyes. It made me more positive and gave me the belief that I could begin to be 'normal' again. It's funny that the rebuilding of my life started in such simple terms – drinking a beer!

Sometime before this, knowing very little about disability, I had met someone who became a good friend, called Jerry Jones. He told me he'd had a motorbike accident and where the car had hit him on his shoulder it had destroyed all the nerves and left his arm withered. He was in groundworks and had done a bit of work for my company, Ray Edwards Ltd. The job was in Windsor and I can remember Jerry digging this pit ready for some drainage with just one hand. I was in awe – I just couldn't believe how he could do that. The tide had changed so much when he saw me in hospital with my arms and legs taken off. My first visual encounter of Jerry was as a disabled person and it was wonderful to see him to give me a bit of insight into how it is. He has been a true friend ever since.

Eventually the subject of home visits started and my God, going home again, where I had left home as the builder. I had built the extension, done so much to the house and now I was going back a totally different person. The visit was set for me to go back to my home, just for a day visit.

What I didn't realise was that things would change so much. I assumed that everything would be the same. I arrived at the house, and was transferred into the wheelchair from the car because I couldn't do anything. Independence was blown out of the window. I was pushed through the front door. Already I felt resentful – I didn't like being dependent on someone to get me through my own front door!

Suddenly I was in the lounge, but it was different. My bed had been brought down and there was a commode next to it. I wondered what was going on. I didn't want to go to the toilet next to my bed; that's not what you do at home. My house had been turned into my hospital room. My home was not my home. Well, I'm sorry, I couldn't cope with that. I swore, I hated everything about it. This was awful. I asked to be taken back to the sanctuary, or cotton wool, of my hospital bed. It was quite sad really that I thought *This is not right, this is not me any more.* I suppose that was the first image of how I perceived my new life and how people see the disabled person. I only wish they had spoken to me about what I would have liked to have seen. They must have discussed this and thought it was for the best. Why didn't they ask me? I thought to myself that maybe I should have listened to them a bit more. To do what I was being told to do and let people help me. But I couldn't. I wanted to do things myself. I was so frustrated and bitter. I wanted to get back to the hospital as soon as I could. I wanted to get away from the house of memories of what I used to be and what I'd lost.

I was a very angry man. I felt resentful for what my life had now become. I didn't want to be disabled. I didn't want to be in a wheelchair. I wanted my life back. Why had this happened to me? I went back to hospital and just lived each day at a time, hoping it would get better. The only thing keeping me going was my twins. They were the only reason to continue.

Eventually it was time to think of my future again, and I was told I was being transferred to Roehampton. It was probably late April when I was well enough to be transferred to the Douglas Bader unit in Roehampton. All I knew about disability was the famous Douglas Bader, the fighter pilot who lost his legs before World War II, being a prat – doing exercises or acrobatics in an aeroplane. He was the only person I remember in the film *Reach for the Sky* with the actor Kenneth More playing him. That was all I knew about amputees and I was going to relive a lot of his thoughts.

I can picture the day I was moved from Hammersmith Hospital to the Douglas Bader unit. It was kind of a repeat: transferred to a wheelchair and pushed through double doors to the ward. A sea of people were in there, but no quad amputees. People had lost one or both of their arms, people had lost their legs, but no one else had lost all four limbs. I was still the one who was different. I was still the person people looked at. I was taken to a solitary room. I hated it, I hated being on my own. I hated being different. I thought it was wrong. It's funny, you think to yourself *I've just come from hospital where I was on a ward with people, but I didn't know too much about it and now I'm getting better I'm on my own.* I cried and cried and cried. It was my release.

My room door opened and in came someone in a white coat, followed by other people in white coats. They started to talk about me, not to me, just like before. I'd had enough. When were they going to treat me like a person? I told them in a very loud voice to f..k off, which wasn't very nice. I was so sick and tired of not being seen or considered. I was tired of people still talking about me, not TO me. It wasn't helping my recovery at all.

A few minutes later, the consultant, Mr Redhead, came in. He sat on my bed and asked, "What would you like?"

Oh my God, a human being. Someone who recognises I have thoughts and needs.

I said, "Thank you. I don't like being spoken about. I'm 32 years old but now I'm being treated like a number. I'm fearful of the future. It's the fear of the unknown. I'm frightened, very, very frightened."

He was so understanding. He listened. He was such a lovely man. I couldn't believe that a man so high up in his field, such a high profile consultant and very knowledgeable, could be so understanding. He had a good bedside manner which reassured me and made me happy.

He could see I was very distressed so he said to me, "Ray, for God sake, what's the problem?"

"I've lost everything. I can't do anything. I'm not independent. I can't go anywhere, I can't look after myself, I can't dress or eat and when I shit, I can't even wipe my arse!"

"Maybe we can help in one way. What if we got you mobile?"

"How?"

He told me he could get electric motorised chairs and you use a remote control stick. He said that maybe if they put a unit on my stump which has a special holder to hold the remote control, then I could be mobile.

"OK, when will that be done? Weeks?"

"No, within an hour you will be able to move around on your own."

Wow! A light was beginning to show through this darkened tunnel. He really understood. I decided this was the man to whom I could ask the questions that no one else seemed to be able to answer. The questions others shied from.

"Why have you put me in solitary?"

"Well Ray, you are a quad amputee. We have never had a quad amputee, so you are quite rare."

"My wife says that!"

"We are really trying to understand what goes on. Believe me, my team have a big job on their hands."

"Am I a guinea pig?"

"In some ways Ray, you will be a very good guinea pig. You will be able to help the future."

How prophetic! When I look back, this was the first time I had any inclination that I might be able to help others. At the time, it seemed the furthest thing from the truth. All I wanted to do was sort myself out, but I was trying to get my mind around what had happened. I suppose I was still in shock.

As luck would have it, the wheelchair arrived, all ready. It was like having a Formula One car arrive, all ready to drive round the track. Independence was golden. You wouldn't know! To be mobile and be myself was amazing. I didn't know how to use the bloody thing because it was quite fast, but I soon learned. As usual, I thought I would be able to manoeuvre it straight away, but of course I couldn't. It took several attempts to get the hang of steering and, even more important, stopping! But having my independence, being able to get around, was bliss.

The next thing on the list was to get me out of my solitude and into the world of other people. I'm a people person, I love to socialise, so being in what I considered solitary confinement felt unnatural. It wouldn't aid my recovery and it certainly wouldn't improve my mental state. I also needed to see people to get used to their reaction to me. Where better to start than with other amputees?

Mr Redhead recognised this and said, "Come on, we'll get you into a different room."

I was in a two-bed room with Neil. I can remember him distinctly: he was a greengrocer, a bit of a 'Jack the lad', who'd lost one leg. He was Metal Mickey, I was Teddy Bear. We struck up a great friendship, a real comradeship. It was so hard for me and yet he helped me progress to no longer feeling sorry for myself. Days went by and, little by little, we learned to understand disability a bit more. I can truly say there was no other quad amputee to bounce ideas off and help me in my plight. No one to ask, "How is this, what do I do?" I could talk to someone with one leg missing but, quite frankly, I won the jackpot. They only needed a crutch but I needed a lot more than that, and I couldn't use a crutch anyway. I'd never seen anyone without any arms or legs, although I had heard about the children affected by thalidomide in the 60s who were born with deformed hands or stumps. This may sound harsh, but if you are born with a disability you live with it, you know no different, you might even understand it. I'd lived through 32 years as an able-bodied person and then suddenly to lose all of your limbs is incomprehensible. I imagine it's like coming home from a war and I truly understand what all these young soldiers go through coming back from Afghanistan and all the war zones. I take my hat off to them and do I admire them? Yes I do!

I can remember the indignity one day when again, I was a very frustrated quad amputee – the teddy bear just sitting on the bed. I really needed to go to the toilet, an easy task for most people. Even most people with disabilities can get into their wheelchair and go to the toilet, but I couldn't.

I remember ringing the bell and it was visiting time. All I could hear was this Jamaican lady shouting in her loud melodious voice, "Do you want the dumping trolley?"

And of course, the visitors heard her. How embarrassing!

She said very loudly (or so it seemed to me), "Ray, what is it you want?"

"Toilet," I whispered, embarrassed, trying to say it without the whole ward hearing.

"You want a big poo?" I just nodded.

She brought the dumping trolley along, and all I was told was: "Transfer on to the commode and do your business." The visitors were all still there, so she pulled the curtains across. Getting on to the dumping trolley was a feat in itself: I had to be careful not to fall off either the bed or the trolley.

I was so relieved to be able to go, the feelings of motions, a natural thing. It was such a relief. But when you've got people around you, you just hope the perfume isn't too smelly. Unfortunately, that wasn't the case. I couldn't stand it, so I don't know about others… Behind the curtains you can sense something is going on around you, you can feel the tension and hear people saying, "Oh my God, what is that smell?" So embarrassing…

I was still in position on the commode and rang the bell and back came my nurse.

"You've done a BIG poo in the dumping trolley! Let's get you off here."

It felt like she was shouting at the top of her voice. Everyone was listening and while she wiped my bottom she described everything like you might to a child: "Oh it's a bit dirty" and she went on and on, or so it seemed. I just wanted a hole to bury myself in.

When she had finished she announced, "I'm going to get rid of this now, bye-bye. I'll turn back the curtains."

I pleaded with her not to, but that made no difference. I wanted to cry on my own. I was tucked back up in bed and she pulled back the curtains. The embarrassment was plain on my face. The visitors must've thought I was unwell.

That was the last time I ever asked for the dumping trolley. From then on, I did my utmost to use the electric chair to get to the toilet. I would not be degraded like that again.

I wondered how the hell they were going to put limbs on a teddy bear. I knew the hospital in Roehampton was trying to put me back together, but I didn't know how they'd manage to achieve it.

In understanding how I was going to be rebuilt, I needed to understand what they were going to do to me. I talked to the rehab team: the consultant, the prosthetist, the physiotherapists, the occupational therapists, and the psychologists. They are all part of the team. I knew if I worked with them, hopefully one day I would walk out of this hospital.

One of the first people I saw was a prosthetist. Prosthetists design your artificial limb to suit you and then make sure it functions in the best way it can. I had one for my upper body and one for my lower body.

The process started with them taking plaster casts of the remaining part of my existing limbs, or stumps. I thought this was very old-fashioned; the only time I remember seeing plaster of Paris before was when I was in the scouts and I used it to make leaves and footprints! It felt strange to have it wrapped around my leg, especially as I'd never broken a bone.

I was excited at the thought that I would soon be standing on my new legs. Unfortunately I couldn't use one of them. The thinning of the blood and the dialysis still working its way through my system, coupled with the drugs I was on, meant it wasn't healing properly.

Eventually I had my limbs cast and a few days later I came in for a fitting. It felt like putting gloves on my hands and socks on my feet, but these were sockets which went around my residual limbs or stumps.

They asked me what type of fittings I wanted for my upper body. At first I looked at hooks, which reminded me of Captain Hook in *Peter Pan*. It was around the time the film *Hook* with Dustin Hoffman came out, so looking like Hook was all the rage…

I thought this was the way to go – at last I'd be able to do something, however small. The arms would be made with hooks at the end and you have straps which go around your back to open and close the limb. You push your arm forward and the strap pulls the hook open and the opposite to close it. You do end up looking a bit like a robot. I have a carbon-fibre grip now, which is more pleasing to the eye.

Self-perception is very important. If you don't like yourself it's hard for the general public, or even your family, to accept what you look like. I gave up looking at myself because I had to move on from that dark place and try to accept what I had become.

When you lose your hands you also lose your dexterity. We depend on these digits to help us do things and no one ever imagines what it is like to be without them. My independence was starting to come back as I began training on how to work my new 'arms'. I was able to use my arm with training and could pick things up. I could finally start to do things for myself, rather than waiting for someone else. Despite this, dressing was out of the question. I couldn't dress myself and being a grown man unable to dress myself was terrible. I couldn't wash myself properly, but I knew it might take many years to understand how I could cope with all this newly built adaptation. At least now I could drink and pick up things.

Once I had my new arms, I went to get my legs. It was mostly the same as before. They fitted the legs to my stumps, but I had something new to contend with: my legs had to bear my weight. I was going to be standing on sticks and what I had left of my original legs was going to have to take all the weight.

I remember the first time I stood up, after months of sitting or lying down. My balance was a bit dodgy, but the adrenaline was pumping. It was like being reborn. I cried, both in pain and in joy. I was in a type of walking area; there were rails on either side and it was like a starting gate at the beginning of a race. I was very frightened and pretty apprehensive. The first step! But eventually I did it and my physios and occupational therapists were by my side, urging me on and praising me. A quad amputee was very rare in those days and the specialists wanted to succeed too.

It must have been frightening for those people to have to rebuild Ray Edwards. How to cope with it? I was such an independent person and now I'd lost my independence, I felt like I'd lost Ray Edwards. My dad had always been my inner strength. I thought about how proud he'd be of me if I could walk out of there.

When I was being fitted for my legs I was asked how tall I was before the amputations. When I came into the hospital, before they removed my legs, I was about five foot five, but I told the doctors I was five foot eight, nearly five foot nine. I thought I could at least gain something from this and I am still that height today! If you want to be taller, make sure you have your legs taken off and then you can be whatever height you want! I wouldn't really recommend it as a way to grow though…

The problem was, because I was taller, my knees were higher and I couldn't get up very easily – I got stuck on a lot of sofas. The bonus was I could see more. It was also strange because I could have any size feet I wanted – my original shoe size didn't matter. I chose size nine. I had great fun going to buy new shoes; the shop assistants would ask if I wanted to try the shoes on. My answer was, "No, I'll put them on my legs and pick them up later."

Finally fitted with the robotic arms and legs, I began to take the first, then second steps. I wanted to get out of those parallel bars, but they wouldn't let me until they could be sure I was safe. There is a lot of work that goes on behind the scenes to get everything right.

It made me so proud to think that I'd mastered the art of standing up and walking again. But you really don't know what life is going to be like when you've got the cotton wool effect from the hospital.

Roehampton Hospital, and the Douglas Bader unit in particular, was kind of like the new parents' home. It was the anchor and I often felt very secure and didn't want to go outside. It was like leaving my home. I know it seems silly, but at any age when you become an amputee it's so frightening, and tears were very much a daily routine because I was so frustrated.

When they eventually got my legs worked out, I couldn't put them on myself and I was worried that I would need help all the time. How would I cope with that? My wife and I were not in a happy place, because of my attitude I think. I was building barriers as a coping mechanism. I wish to God I had understood more at that time, but mostly I just wanted to die.

For my twins' sake I wanted to be able to walk out of the unit and stand with them and cuddle them as best I could. To say, "Here's your dad." At this time, I still couldn't dress and I couldn't do much at all. The idea of the two appendages on my upper arms was beginning to wear me out. I found it difficult to use both hooks, mainly because I'd lost a lot more of my arm on the left side than the right, so my right arm dominates. I decided just to use the right arm as my dominant arm and asked the prosthetist to build me a merely cosmetic arm for my left. It didn't do anything, but it gave me balance and it looked better. Even today, this is how I am and by doing this I could concentrate more on successfully using my right arm.

I assumed I would always need a wheelchair, but I was determined to succeed with learning to walk again. I used to read *Reach for the Sky* about Douglas Bader and that kept me determined; he was so determined he made his stumps bleed, and I was sure I was on the same trajectory. Standing next to the electric wheelchair that had given me my first taste of independence and activity was a really good feeling. What a long journey I'd had in such a short space of time!

It was a huge learning curve understanding how to wear the limbs and it did hurt. The stumps were still a bit sore, they were swollen, and the attachments were Velcro straps. We knew that every so often we'd have to renew the limbs.

So I was in the famous Douglas Bader unit, the icon I had to live up to. It's funny, when you come out of your room and you sit around the table, sitting in the electric wheelchair, you look at people and you get friendly. There were elderly people, women, all different types. There was a lovely lady called Louise. She'd had a motorbike accident. She came in very soon after I did and we had a great friendship. We took the mickey out of each other. When you take the mickey out of each other in a place like that, black humour doesn't matter. You get legless, you really do. It is just a funny thing. What I didn't like were the condescending people like the occupational therapists. I remember one telling me that today we were going to make a toilet roll holder.

"No we're bloody not. As a builder I normally go and buy one. There is no way on earth I'm going to make a toilet roll holder."

Louise and I both hated the condescending way we were treated by some people, so we decided to get our own back. We saw there was a room where you could learn to make things and models. One day, we got hold of some plasticine and made a model of a phallic symbol which we stuck to the occupational therapist's chair! We wanted to give her a message. I don't know what she thought of it or if she knew who'd done it, but I suspect she did.

So we did have fun at times. We were making the best of the whole situation. You have to be strong and when you've been through a trauma, you use that strength in whatever way you can.

While I was in the unit, I spied a computer at the back of the room and asked if I could be taught to use it. I was told it would be fine, so I started to learn how to work it. I hadn't been brought up with computers, or even calculators, the only thing we had was a slide rule, so I was intrigued by this computer. It was such an old thing it was run on steam: if you switched it on in the morning, it was ready to use mid-afternoon. But I was able to tap things out. Wow! Not only could I now walk, I could start to do things myself. I thought about my building company and wondered if I could do quotes. It was the start of a rebuilding curve and it was brilliant being able to do even small things again.

Now I had my arms and legs, I wanted to do more. I wanted to get back to real life, so I did have trips home again. It wasn't an easy time, but at least this time I walked through the front door. I was able to stay. Maybe it was easier because I knew what to expect. But it still wasn't easy. I still couldn't climb stairs very easily, and that was another thing I wanted to conquer. I was sleeping downstairs and I missed the cuddles with my wife and with my children, but at least I was able to have a life at home for a bit and then return to the hospital for my therapies. It provided me comfort and it was good fun.

I asked my dad if I'd ever go home permanently. The twins were getting older and of course I knew June 4th, their first birthday, was getting closer. How would I see them? Would I be home?

A few days before their birthday, I was getting quite good on my limbs and so more independent. A bit cocky really. I'd become quite famous because the quad amputee had risen! I was the bionic man! I really fancied a beer. A few of us thought *Why don't we get some taxis and go down the pub?*

The pub was called The Montague Arms in Roehampton Lane. It was a beautiful warm evening, the taxis were waiting. I had all the limbs on. I was wearing a short-sleeved shirt, as it was warm, and trousers, quite smart really. A few of us were going. Neil didn't wear his limb, so he was hopping. It was a Metal Mickeys reunion. I was a bit of a pillock because I hadn't had a good beer for a couple of months. When I was a builder I'd always call into the pub when finishing, but I'd been in hospital for nearly three months and, apart from the beer Dad brought me in Hammersmith Hospital, not a drop had passed my lips. I hadn't thought about not being able to drink like I could before, all I was focused on was having a drink. Being normal!

I think the landlord was thinking it was going to be an easy night: mid-week, not a lot going on. How wrong he was!

He opened the pub and in flew a group of Metal Mickeys, hobbling down the steps into the bar. He looked surprised.

We were all enjoying the release from the hospital environment – both the drink and the freedom. Several pints later, I was drinking away, beginning to forget the situation I was in. Beginning to forget everything. But we hadn't really thought about going to the toilet or about the fact that when you've drunk alcohol you tend to go to the toilet more. I asked the landlord where the toilet was and he told me it was down the steps. When he spoke those words 'down the steps' I thought *Oh God, the war-zone. What are we going to do?*

I hadn't mastered stairs yet so Neil offered to come with me. "How can you? You're hobbling," I said. But Neil insisted and I suppose I thought there was safety in numbers.

I took the steps very carefully, but beer in, brain out, you don't care what happens. I eventually got to the toilet, oh the relief! I hadn't really learned how to use the hook properly, so splashed everywhere, but at least there was relief somehow. We walked back. All OK. Now we had done this once, we were confident it would be fine every time. This happened on numerous occasions during the evening. It got more and more difficult as the beer flowed and we lost our inhibitions, but who cared? We were enjoying ourselves. By the end of the evening, it was more a fall down the stairs to the toilet rather than a hobble.

The nursing sister had given us a curfew of 11pm. At 11.30 we arrived back, after many pints, a little bit drunk because we didn't know how little we could drink. Maybe that should be 'a lot drunk' although we didn't realise this. Being cocky now, we ended up outside the ward and we knew there were tables and chairs there. We all sat down and the nurses were with us, drinking and talking. Unfortunately I thought I was on a building site – I was reliving the old Ray Edwards – so instead of finding the toilet in the ward, I went round the side of the building. I was very unstable on my artificial legs and as I went to go to the toilet I tripped into a rose bush. By now, I had got hold of my penis and was crushing it. I was so drunk and disorientated I didn't know what to do. I couldn't work out how to work my arm or what to do. I couldn't get up on my own, so there I was in the rose bush, wanting to go to the toilet but quite stuck!

I heard the sound of crutches and it was Neil.

"Ray, where are you?"

Of course, I was down on the ground in the rose bush.

"What are you doing down there?"

I said I was just thinking I was on a building site and the next thing I knew he was in the rose bush too!

He had fallen over and was also stuck. So there we were, both of us on the ground, in the rose bush, me still desperate to go to the toilet and neither of us able to move!

The nurses came to pick us up, Neil and I relieved ourselves and we returned – a little bit bruised, but feeling better. We finished our beer and went to bed. I should say eventually we got to bed – neither of us could manage that without help. I don't know how I got to bed, or who put me in bed, but I know when I woke up in the morning my arms and legs were all over the place across the floor. I don't remember much!

The next day I had a splitting headache. I was woken up at 6am – a stupid time to be woken up – and my electric wheelchair was by the side of my bed.

"Ray, you need to get up."

"No, I have a headache."

"Put your underpants on and get in the wheelchair. You need to get up. Sister is annoyed, she's going to give you a talking to. You're a disgrace, you've led the men astray. Some of them were sick, it's terrible."

Neil and I looked at each other.

"What bullshit and bollocks. We need to get out of here."

We went to have breakfast and unsurprisingly my head was throbbing. I think all the other guys were suffering too. I thought now I'd had a bit of breakfast I'd have a shower and a shave. I knew the Commandant (as we called the sister) wanted to see us, but I didn't care. I thought I'd go to see her before she came to see me to give me a telling-off.

I tried to explain. "I'll tell you what – before you talk to me I'll talk to you. Maybe we shouldn't have done what we did but what a great night and it showed that we're people, human beings. Quite honestly, I think I've had enough of this place, so I'm going to discharge myself.

You can tell me what you want, you can tell me off, but that is what I'm doing."

I think she was surprised to have someone standing up to her, but I didn't care.

Everyone knew my twins' birthday was coming up and I walked out of hospital on their first birthday – 4th June 1987. I was as proud as Punch. I hear now that they don't allow alcohol any more and I wonder if that was my doing, but hey ho, it gave me the nudge I needed and I am glad I did it.

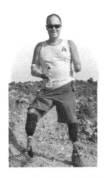

CHAPTER FOUR

The Builder re-built

When I did eventually get on my legs and walk out of the hospital, after being a bit of a boy the night before, it was a tough call to go home and, as I said, I was not the same person. Whatever I did I was going to cause trouble really. I wanted it to be the same, but it wasn't.

Arriving home from the cotton wool environment of the Douglas Bader unit on my children's first birthday – well, the excitement, so many emotions. Fear of the unknown, tears running down my face as we got home and even now I can remember it was so emotional to go through the front door, to WALK through the front door, thinking *Here we go!* I had learned to walk up and down stairs so my house had become my home again.

But Ray Edwards was not Ray Edwards. He was not the same man who left and now he had been rebuilt with arms and legs. How would I cope?

A party had been arranged, I do not know by whom, to celebrate my home-coming. It was great to have the party, with everyone there, seeing the family again. I know it was done with the best of intentions and I suppose in my own mind I was conscious that outwardly I was really an OK person. With these adapted limbs, no one would know I was any different, apart from the hook and the artificial hand, and with trousers on, no one knew. But how was the mind? How was I personally going to cope? What did people think of me? How did I want to be perceived and what did I think of myself? How was I going to cope with being disabled? I couldn't do anything manually.

In the early days, when I came back from hospital, the twins were just one year old. How would they approach me, as their dad? Would they notice any difference? I remember being on my knees a lot with them, and when they were in their cots, I can remember them being so close to me. As I had no hands to hold their little hands, I managed to put my stump through the rails on the cots. They could then cuddle my arm, but it was not the same. Was it the same for them? Did they understand this was my way of having physical contact? As I say, these were the early days. I loved my children dearly and when I was on my knees I could wander around, look after them and play with them, in the garden as well. Bath time was great, as they would be in the bath with me, with my wife supervising. Looking back, I think I didn't realise how they would help me in the learning process of dealing with my disability.

The days went into months and I found it so frustrating, living as an amputee. I hated the loss of my independence.

I hated having to ask people to do things for me, or waiting for them to do things. I hated being reliant on anyone or anything. I also hated not being able to work in the same way I did before. I am a very active person and I felt trapped, because every time I wanted to do something it took so much effort, organisation and usually someone else to help me. But most of all I hated me, because I was not me! No one understood what life was about. I needed a release and I think drink was kind of a solace, a break from the norm for me.

A couple of drinks turned into more drinks which turned into even more drinks, to cover up my frustration and really my hatred of myself. I had built a wall around me, and no one was going to penetrate that. My dad was a strong character, and it was inbuilt in me to be like him but I don't think even Dad realised how strong you would have to be to cope with all I had gone through. All I wanted was to be loved like the old Ray was. I wanted to be me. But you can't ask for things and you can't dictate how people will perceive you. If you don't like yourself, you are not oozing out anything to others to like you, to reciprocate. My way of life did not make people say 'we love you'. If you are a happy person, then your life around you is happy. If you are miserable, then life is miserable around you. Until I could come to terms with this, nothing would change.

My wife had been through so much and had to carry on with life, looking after the twins, and now she had another baby to look after: me. It was very hard for her and I did not make it any easier.

Maybe six months down the line, when things were not happy at home, we thought maybe a break would be a good idea, for me to go away on holiday. It was a frightening thought, to go away from the world I was familiar with. It was a huge thing to contemplate but my dear friend Jerry said he would go with me. Bless him, he has one arm, could he cope with me? But I had known him for a long, long time and I thought it would be fine. I don't think he realised what he was taking on and I certainly didn't understand the complications of travelling abroad being disabled. All I could think about was being away – away from the environment I called home and away from everyone feeling sorry for me. I thought I could escape. But escape from what? I think it was a good learning curve for me.

We ended up in Malta for two weeks. Oh my God, it was like two boys in a sweet shop! We had so much fun. I hadn't got swimming legs and I was not capable of doing things I can do now, but it was still a break for me, away from what was now 'normal' life. The sheer friendship and kindness from Jerry was so rewarding and so needed at the time. But then of course my jealous side came in, thinking about my wife having the twins on her own, being with the family, and I couldn't understand why I could not be with my wife. Why did I have to do things on my own? Why was my marriage not working?

In the evening at the hotel, I was hitting the booze and that made me more depressed. But overall, the two weeks was a break from everybody. I thank Jerry from the bottom of my heart for making it happen. We bonded very well as dear friends and we met so many people. We did a lot of things, had evenings out and we even met with some disabled people in a bar one night. It was just like watching Metal Mickeys in a bar, getting drunk. It was so funny. There was myself with four limbs missing, Jerry with one arm missing, another guy with one arm, a guy with one eye and another in a wheelchair. We just chilled out. It was a very, very funny evening. Mind you, we woke up with headaches the next morning, but that was the way it was really. It was like an old-fashioned 18-30s holiday, I call it. Great!

Returning home only brought back all the problems I had before I went away. One of the big problems I needed to sort was what was I to do for work?

I still had Ray Edwards Ltd, so I decided once I had learned to use the computer that I could use the log cabin in my garden as the office.

One of the problems I had was being able to get around. I was used to driving myself everywhere and now I could not. I was quite a good driver, I had my HGV licence and could drive anything. How was I to drive with no arms or legs? I knew people had adaptations put into cars, but would that be possible for me? Also, I had to pass a test to prove I was able to drive. This was degrading, as I had been driving for many years and I loved my cars. Cars were part of me, so why did I have to prove I could drive?

Well, I bit the bullet and decided that if I could have a car adapted and prove I could drive, then this would aid my mobility even more. So I went to Banstead mobility centre, near Carshalton, with my consultant Dr Soori, my wife and a few others. I loved cars and loved driving and in my mind I was the same driver, but of course, having no limbs, this was a bit of a silly statement. The cocksure me, at 32 years old, said I could drive anything. So they told me to get into the adapted car and try. They got into the car with me, a silly thing to do really, especially with the attitude I had.

I had split hooks in those days, so I looked like Captain Hook, and of course my artificial legs. I started up the car, no problem, started off, OK so far and then as I began to accelerate, I did not have the dexterity to put the accelerator pedal down slowly, so I sped off and then braked hard, again due to lack of feeling in my limbs. The people in the back of the car nearly ended up in the front and the doctor almost went through the windscreen.

They said, "Ray, get out of the bloody car because you are going to kill someone. Let's go to the simulator."

I had to concede this was the best option, as I realised this was the only way I could learn to drive as a quad amputee and no one would allow me near a car if I did not.

Remember, this was 1987, so it was not as modern as it is these days, and it was a simulator of a Cortina. Not my kind of car, but I could not choose what I wanted. I was told to sit in the driving seat and act as if I was going to drive. I put pressure on the accelerator and the brake with my right foot and tried to move the steering wheel with my hooks. Not an easy task. I had to be taught how to use my artificial limbs to drive the car. So soul destroying…

However, it taught me a lesson. I really wasn't able to drive at that time and from now on I would have to learn to do everything over again. There was nothing I could take for granted any more. Gone were all my skills and abilities. I was like a child learning to do everything for the first time. I never thought about this before my operations and it is so important for me now to give out information to others. I persevered and then was able to pass certain standards, so I could drive my car. Luckily it needed very little adaptation: just a unit on the steering wheel, to use with my artificial limbs. It gave me my mobility and I was able to go from Banstead with a passing-out certificate, able to drive again.

Things were better for a time now I was more mobile. It got me out from worrying about myself. I was able to drive again, which was really important to me. Unfortunately, the car I had adapted was an Escort, but they adapted it in such a way that although it had been automatic and I could use the pedals with my feet, I found visually it wasn't a car that I liked to drive very much. It didn't go with the Ray Edwards image of old! But it gave me the independence: I was able to go out and do my normal day's work, measuring jobs. I still kept my subcontractors working with me, and in some ways I felt as though I was back to a normal working life.

But inside I was being eaten away, not being able to do what I used to be able to do. I didn't realise that I wouldn't be able to dress myself, I couldn't even wash myself in those days. The teddy bear syndrome was there, no arms and legs, just sat there, it's not very nice.

Unfortunately, the drink did get to me, we kept arguing, my wife and I, and it wasn't very good for the whole atmosphere of the house. We had a chance to move from this particular house, to find a bungalow with land. We moved and I think that was probably the downfall; I shouldn't have done that. The bungalow needed a lot of work doing to it and although I had the construction company, I don't think I realised how hard it would be. When you are arguing all the time, you are not clear and understanding. We lived separate lives really and it was just awful. I don't think I was a very good provider, I don't think I was a very good dad. I was so horrible to everyone; I was hell and drink took over me. I do remember the one time when I did a successful job, and it brought in quite a nice profit. I loved Jaguars and I was able to go out and buy a 3.4 Jaguar in Weybridge. I was so proud. The small adaptation I made was a steering unit; my right hook around the steering wheel gave me a sense of independence. I thought *Ray, you have done it again!* So I had my own number plate and car, but it didn't really bring happiness. All I wanted was to be loved and be the old Ray again. They do say you can't buy health and you can't buy happiness. I was trying to buy happiness and that wasn't working. It was so bad that I although I was working hard, I wasn't a happy man. I realised that I had got to change.

Unfortunately my wife and I decided the marriage was not going to work; I couldn't cope with it and I had pushed her away by now. I think it was very tough for her to cope with the twins and me. I was no fun at all and it must have been miserable for her. It got so bad that there was a period when I lost the plot and drank and drank to take away the inner pain. I used to phone my mum and dad telling them how unhappy I was. I don't know what I expected them to do but they were the only people I could talk to.

One day I was in the pub, drunk again. I got in the car and I was really over the limit. I drove the Jaguar into a little lane and I sat there looking at the moonlit sky, at the stars. It was a lovely clear evening and I could see a big oak tree at the end of the lane. Tears were rolling down my face. I had really got to the end of the line. All I wanted to be was me. I wanted to go home and my wife to give me a cuddle just like normal people do. But it seemed my life was a pattern of war: I finished one war zone, came home and found I was going into another one. That was about it. I couldn't cope any more. I knew I had a family, but that wasn't enough.

I started up the car, revved it up and put my foot down hard on the accelerator, heading straight for the tree. It was a bloody big tree, this oak tree. I can remember it looming up very quick and in a split second the car hit this damn tree. Oak trees and cars are different materials and this oak tree had been there hundreds of years and it was not going to be moved by a Jaguar. The Jaguar came off a bit the worse for wear, and thank goodness I was so full of alcohol and supple, because the door fell open and I fell out to the side of it. I did have my seatbelt on, but there was enough play in it that I fell out. So, even trying to do that I couldn't do it right…

In the last chapter I recounted the vision I had in the chapel at Roehampton, of my guardian angel. In a spilt second I thought *That guardian angel, the bugger won't let me go at all!* I looked up and it was such a clear sky. The moon was bright and the stars were shining. I thought *You are a silly bloody idiot Ray.*

Tears were streaming down my face by now. I wasn't hurt physically, but mentally I had done more damage than I thought. Why? My twins needed their daddy, I was their daddy. What was I doing? This was a private road where I had hit the tree and luckily enough there was a house nearby.

The people came out and said, "Are you all right?"

I was a very lucky man in that I didn't have to worry about the police and everything. The people had not called them and as I just got up, they asked me if I was all right, and I said no.

I don't know why they did not call the police, maybe they were in shock at seeing this mangled car, totally wrecked, and a drunk man with false arms just pick himself up and walk away. Maybe they were scared. Who knows?

I knew where the pub was, a mile down the road. I left the car there and walked back. I knew a chap who had a garage and I would get him to pick it up. I walked back to the pub, had a few more drinks and got a taxi home. I think the moral of this story is that there was no way Ray was ready to leave this mortal coil. It dawned on me I was a silly sod and that drink was not doing me any good at all. I just had to pack it in and accept, if I could, what I had got left. I know you always look around and people are worse off than you and I felt there was something above, looking after me. I also thought about all the people who had looked after me: my family, friends and the teams of people at Roehampton and Hammersmith – everyone who had looked after me so far. They are my reason for doing things. It would be nice to say thank you very much, I can now get on with my life. I realised I had been very selfish and should start to think about other people. The world did not revolve around me. The twins needed their daddy. From this moment I tried to turn my life around a bit.

My brother knew what had happened to my car so he was good enough to lend me his car. It was a kind gesture and I liked being looked after by my parents again for a while. They really, really looked after me. But I still liked to drink now and again.

I was not in a very good place with my wife then and so we decided to split up. I was so unhappy but I didn't want to show my feelings to my children. I would lean my head against the cot rails, look at the children, and when they were up, I would sit with them on the floor. I was like a baby as well. They would cuddle me. It was the closest I could get to being a hands-on dad, excuse the pun! I was very much in love with them and I was still in love with my wife then, but I just couldn't get anything right. I had this feeling that things would get worse if we stayed together. My twins were my saviour. We used to play a lot. I used to try to do things the best I could, I loved being with them when I could. But it was a very, very volatile situation, so unhappy, and I did not want them to be the pawn in the chess game. My wife had to decide what to do. We both knew it was the right thing to split up and of course she had the children because I struggled to look after myself, let alone them. But it was tough seeing them just now and again, and even to this day I regret that I missed being with them growing up and I feel as if I was never a dad to them. If I could ever put that right, put the milk back in the bottle, I would.

It was too late to stop the divorce and everything. I just had to maintain my own life. So what could I do?

Well, I had two thoughts: I had to leave the marital home, and go back to live with my mum and dad for a while. They lived in Wentworth, a smart area, and Dad was semi-retired but together with my brother, they were still running Edwards Construction. Going home to my mum and dad's at the age of 32/33 was not a very nice thought, but then you only have one mum and dad and they will always love you. Blood is thicker than water.

I have always strived to have as much dexterity as possible, so if there was a new type of limb produced, I would want to try it. In the days when I was still getting used to artificial limbs I heard about a new electric limb, called the MYO electric. I asked about this and found there was a possibility for me to be able to wear one of these. It was a carbon-fibre or a hook that worked by electric motors. There are sensors put on your arm or the stump where the muscles react and open and close this particular hook. I managed to work it all out and the powers that be produced quite a modern-looking hook that worked by my muscle impulse.

It meant I was able to drive more easily with this and so my friend and I went out for a drive to test it out. All was going well and we ended up at a pub, of course. The pub was The Foresters in Ascot. This hook was fantastic: it had given me much more dexterity but I had only used it so far for driving. Going into the pub, I ordered a pint, great success, much easier to drink with my new hand. After having drunk nearly a pint I needed to go to the toilet. Now, my brain wasn't really working. I walked into the toilet and there was a man already in there. We had a chat, as men do, standing in front of the urinal. As I was chatting I opened the zip with my artificial hook and eased my precious manhood out, and once I got ready to do the business a noise came from nowhere. It was the battery enclosure for the motor of the arm and it was a kind of a dying whirring sound. Unfortunately I captured my little manhood in my gripper as the battery died! The pain was excruciating. Tears ran down my face. I could not move. I could not release the grip, as the battery was dead and I had no way of moving or controlling the pain. Added to this, I still needed to pass water.

Luckily the man was still standing next to me, so I squeaked at him, as best I could, to get help. I told him there was someone at the bar who knew me, so please could he go and get him to help. He said nothing, just ran out of the door, which was near to where I was standing.

I could hear him shout, "Does anyone know a person who has an artificial hook because he has it stuck around his…" Use your own imagination for the word he used. The panic was then transferred to the pub and everyone looked around, obviously wondering who it could be. My friend had to leave his drink, stand up in front of everyone in the pub and walk into the toilet to help me. The embarrassment for both of us was overwhelming.

The battery had died, however I had a spare battery in my coat pocket and my friend then had to take out the old battery and replace the new one, while my hook was still in the position it had come to a halt in. Of course, this is quite difficult to do in that situation, so although the battery was in the enclosure, it was not locked tight. Neither of us realised this, as we were just relieved to have sorted the situation. I know I was more relieved than him, in many ways! I put a brave face on it but I was in agony. My manhood was throbbing, I didn't feel very well and could not walk properly. I knew that when we walked out of the toilet everyone would be looking at us, but we both held our heads up high and walked back to the bar. I thought the situation was over, except for the pain and swelling, but how wrong could I have been! I could feel eyes in the back of my head, but took no notice as the hook opened and I grabbed my glass to finish my drink. Unfortunately, as I picked up the glass I felt something leave my arm, but did not know it was the battery coming out of the enclosure. I was still in pain, throbbing away and all I could see was a bullet (the battery) flying towards the back of the bar! The back of the bar was a mirror and this 'bullet' was flying towards it. In a split second there was a crash on the floor and the mirror was shattered. Completely broken! Now, I was still in pain, I couldn't release the pint glass out of my hook because the arm had seized up as the battery was not there, and the mirror was in pieces and the optics were also broken, due to the mirror breaking.

The landlord came up to me and said, "Look, I have heard you have hurt yourself down below, but you didn't have to come out and break up my bloody pub!"

All I could say was, "Please may I have my battery back?"

He was very kind, he gave it back to me and then told me to go and not to come back again and I have never been back since.

One time, I walked out of the pub, really the worse for wear, and opposite the pub was a little path and a stream. This stream is dry until it gets flooded from the rain. How I did it, I don't know, but I ended up in the stream. When I stood up, my head was just above road level. It was just becoming dark, so the light was fading. Cars were going past and there was this village idiot, walking down the stream with artificial arms and legs! It was getting darker and darker and I remembered I had my phone so I used the light from my phone to see where I was going. Now, as I lacked dexterity due to no fingers, I had to poke the buttons to make the phone light up, to use as a torch. I was struggling to keep the light on. I became aware of someone in a car slowing up. They must have seen this idiot in the ditch, but they didn't stop. They revved up and sped off. They must have called the police because in the next few minutes I heard a siren. A police car arrived and a policeman got out. I suppose I was quite a funny sight. A drunk in a ditch, and a quad amputee at that!

This young policeman looked down at me and said, "What are you doing in the ditch?"

In my slurred way, I replied, "I don't know." It was a comedy sketch really. It was just so funny.

He said, "How did you get down there?"

Again I said, "I don't know."

"Where are you going?"

"For a drink." And that was what I kept saying: "For a drink, I am going to the pub just up the road."

"What are you doing in the ditch?"

"I don't know."

In the end he said, "Let's help you out."

So he helped me out and looked at me and asked me what had happened to me. I explained I had no arms or legs and I was going through a divorce and I was not happy and that type of thing so he then asked me where I lived. Well, when you find an idiot in a ditch, and you ask them where they live, if they said Wentworth, you would think *You are having a joke* because Wentworth is posh. But my mum and dad did live in Wentworth. I gave him the address and he said he would take me home. He told me to sit in the back of the car, but I said I couldn't because I couldn't get in due to having no arms or legs. So he helped me into the front and he became my chauffeur for the night. He was a really nice guy. He could have been quite angry with me.

As I sat in the front of the car I said, "As you are going to Egham, you could take me home, it is not very far away."

So he did.

As we got nearer I said, "Please don't take the car into the drive, I don't want the neighbours to see me getting out of a police car."

So he dropped me nearby. As I was getting out of the car I said, "Thank you very much indeed. Look, I am going to the pub tomorrow. Can you pick me up?"

Laughing he said, "Ray, no more!"

That was my attention from the law that day and the next morning I told my dad. He said, "You are an idiot!" Dad dropped some cash into the police charity to say thank you.

That was one of my brushes with the police, due to being silly. It is quite entertaining, but hey ho!

Eventually the divorce came through and I decided I needed a place of my own so I ended up in a one-bedroomed flat at Addlestone. My wife had the children and I really had lost the lot.

I knew I had to start to live my life again. I carried on drinking and used to visit another couple of pubs on a very regular basis. Every time I went out, no matter with whom or where I was going, I seemed to end up in a pub. There was a lady in one of the pubs who was often there and she took a liking to me. I was not in the right frame of mind. I didn't care, but we got to know each other. A goes to B, B goes to C and suddenly she is pregnant! She was rather nice, she looked after me, but I couldn't cope with too much affection. I just couldn't cope. I was lost in the wilderness, but hey ho, something was working!

Looking back, I had so much trouble with my wife conceiving children; because of the cancer treatment, they said I had no bullets firing, then suddenly you lose your arms and legs, you have a new gun and there are many bullets! I thought *Never, in my dreams!* It was not a case of going with every girl and being a ram, because I am not like that, but it was just astonishing, and quite a shock. At that particular time, I wasn't out to upset anybody and this young girl was a very, very caring person. She showed me kindness, love and affection. That was what I was craving for, because I just didn't know what to do. I am a human being, albeit a teddy bear, and we all need love. A teddy bear is cuddly. Christopher was born on Christmas Day. I was quite proud really. I remember seeing him the next day. Unfortunately, I was not in the right frame of mind or in the right place to cope with it. His mother and I parted. It was probably my fault and I feel very guilty about it. I don't know what else to say. That part of my life was very tough to cope with.

The last straw basically was driving my brother's car from the pub and unfortunately I lost control. I crashed into a shop window. The police were called again and this time I was taken to the police station and was done for drink-driving. I had now completely ruined my life. I had ended up in this one-bedroomed flat, unable to drive, a very unhappy man. Believe me, when you are in a situation where things seem hopeless and you feel no one loves you, it is a horrible situation.

Mum and Dad would come over now and then. When you ask people for things, it is very hard, because you are not independent. I had lost my independence with the loss of my arms and legs and now I had lost my main mobility. I was 12 months without my licence. I said to Dad, "I can't cope with this. I still have a business to run and I can't do it. I am a nothing. I am a complete nothing."

There was a light in the tunnel. I was due to meet the angel who turned my life around…

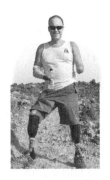

CHAPTER FIVE

My Guardian Angel

Dad used to say to me, "Don't worry son, you never have to play on your own. Don't despair, things will happen for a reason and you never know, there might be a silver lining." How right he was!

Dad and I were invited to a retirement do for the bank manager of the Nat West in Egham. We both knew him, as we both used the same bank. The event took place at Holloway College on Egham Hill, near the green. At this time I still couldn't drive because of my drink-driving ban, so Dad was the driver. I wanted to go because it gave me an excuse to dress up and, of course, there would be free-flowing drink there. A chance to enjoy myself.

The event was in the picture gallery at the college and my God, what a beautiful building. A room full of Monets, Constables, you name it – I had never seen such beautiful paintings. I had never been in such an exquisite place.

"Marvellous," I said to Dad. "Take some of these off the wall, we could make a fortune."

It was a lovely evening, meeting and greeting, and I met the staff of the Nat West. I had been into the bank before, but that was before I had my accident; now I was testing how people would react to me. Would they be different? I had got to know some of the staff and they were always friendly, and they still were tonight. I always made friends easily.

The evening was great. I was drinking with everyone and how quickly the time passed and it was time to go. Time to say our farewells to the manager and his staff.

There was one particular young lady, Fiona, who I didn't really know, but she knew me. I think my reputation had gone before me and word had got round about what had happened to me, so she probably felt she knew me already. I had probably met her before, but didn't remember.

A few of the girls, including Fiona, said they were going to the Red Lion in Egham, as the night was still young. Well, pub, Ray, the two go together like bread and butter. I was enjoying myself too much for the evening to end and if the chance of drink is around, I'm there. We go together well.

I wasn't backward in coming forward, so without an invitation I said, "I'm up for that. Can I have a lift?"

Fiona had her car and so I looked her straight in the eye when I asked the question, hoping she would say I could go with her. I didn't even consider what she wanted or thought, I just asked her to give me a lift. I know I was a bit forward, but so what. Luckily she agreed to give me a lift so off we went. I sat in the front of the car because I couldn't get in the back; a couple of her friends sat in the back. When we got to the Red Lion I carried on drinking and talking, having a really good time. Fiona and I spent most of the evening just chatting to each other and it was only later we realised everyone had disappeared. They had gone home, I think. We didn't care. The two of us were alone, chatting and enjoying each other's company.

We hadn't had anything to eat, which we suddenly realised now we were alone, and so I didn't ask her out or anything, we just decided it was time to eat and left the pub in search of food. We ended up going out for dinner. We had a curry and just talked and talked. She was a very good listener. I talked like I had never talked before. I could tell her things and she understood. She didn't judge or comment, she just listened. She was such a lovely person to be with. The time was getting late and so I told her I had to go home. She asked if I had a car, I told her no, but I didn't tell her I had lost my licence. I was too embarrassed – after all, I was trying to make a good impression. I thought I would tell her that later, when I had got to know her better.

We decided to meet a few days later. It was one of those odd things, how we met and bonded. We continued to meet more and more, that evolved and we became very good friends. She really is a diamond lady, so lovely. She sees me as me, not a teddy bear. She is with me for who I am, not what I am. She has a great sense of humour and she certainly is a character. We got to know each other very well and then I moved into her place in Staines. It made sense. We were together so much and it seemed silly to have two places and she could also look after me and care for me. We became very close.

I explained after a time that I had lost my licence. She asked me what else had happened. My reputation seemed to have gone before me. She knew I liked a drink or two and I did booze a bit, well a lot really. I had always liked a drink and since the accident drink had been my release, my solace, my way of coping. Fiona didn't really like the amount I drank, but she put up with it; I think she just accepted why I drank. Meeting Fiona was a breath of fresh air, but my God, didn't she go through the mill with me! She was so patient. I would regularly go drinking and she would wait for me outside the pub or the club to take me home. Sometimes she would get annoyed, but she had the patience of a saint. How she stood by me, I don't know; I was really a pig to her. My love goes to her and always will and I thank her so much for staying with me. Bless her.

It came to a head one night not long after I had moved into her place in Staines. I had gone out with friends and done my usual: won't be long, just a couple. I ended up coming home late at night, so drunk I fell though her door.

I think by now Fi had got a bit fed up with my drinking and so she tried to curb my ways, make me understand why I drank, and she succeeded. I know she did it because she loves me, she looks after me so well. She is a really good friend, my best friend.

I eventually realised this and so I made a decision to be brave. One day, when I came home I plucked up courage and told her how much I loved her and then asked her to marry me and lo and behold, she said yes! I thought *Oh my God,* I was so surprised. I didn't think she would say yes, even though it was what I wanted. It really boosted my self-esteem.

Although my wife and I had divorced, so there was no problem marrying Fiona, I did have a family already: my twins. Fiona had met my twins and she knew what she was taking on. It is very difficult for a lady to take on another person and his children, let alone a quad amputee and a strong-willed one at that. All I can say is she is amazing to have done that.

On our wedding day, which was wonderful, Dad said in his speech, "Well, one thing in Ray's favour is that God sent an angel down to look after him. Fiona is the angel. I am so pleased."

I think Mum and Dad were so worried about me, being such an independent man and then becoming the teddy bear I was. How would I cope with life? I needed someone to look after me, to make sure I could cope with what life had thrown at me. My guardian angel. There she was: Fiona.

She still has that role now. She puts me together and takes me apart.

I said, "You have your own Action Man. You can put me together and dress me up in any clothes you want. You can even dress me as the Village People." Thank goodness she doesn't, but I do have to keep on the right side of her, just in case.

She has a good sense of humour. We do have some laughs. If you laugh together that is what life is all about. She is my mate, my love, my best friend.

We wanted our own place, one we had bought together. I sold my flat, she sold her house and we bought a three-bedroomed place in Staines. It was a road away from where I lived as a child. How funny to turn it around to be in the area where I was when I was young. Mum and Dad had loved that house and life was great then.

Life was great for Fiona and me too. We were even blessed with children. We had a little girl, Nicola, who was born in Staines. Life was absolutely gorgeous. I got my licence back and I started driving again. I bought a 3-series BMW, which I loved, and I was working for my dad again, helping him, just like old times.

It was the start of recovery, but the old drink still came back. I did need a drink now and again, I don't know why. All I can think is that was the old Ray trying to get out. I was trying to prove nothing had changed and I could still be the person I was. But drink made me not very nice.

I had a horrible attitude and in fact I was a pig! Fiona was very good at coping with me; she knew instinctively what to do. She probably understood more than I did what was going on. At the time I couldn't understand anything at all and was fighting my inner self. My mental state was not good. Bless her, she coped and put up with me. In fact she did more than that, she helped me.

There was one particular time I came home so drunk that I tried to walk upstairs and I fell backwards. How I didn't break my neck I don't know, because remember even when I am sober walking upstairs is not as easy for me as for people with two legs. I landed at the bottom of the stairs in a heap. In the process I had cut my lip and it was bleeding but I didn't even realise, let alone care.

I remember Fiona coming downstairs and saying, "Just put this towel under your head and go to sleep." I ended up sleeping at the bottom of the stairs. I couldn't get upstairs anyway.

The next morning I had to go to do a survey for a contract. I think it was an elderly person wanting an adaptation to the house. I can remember being picked up by one of my subcontractors. He said, "Are you all right Ray?"

I couldn't talk because my lip had swollen and I could only talk with a lisp. He asked me what had happened and I explained. Thank goodness he had picked me up, because I was in no fit state to drive. I had hurt my back as well, so when we arrived at the house I limped in. The gentleman opened the door and I tried to introduce myself, mumbling, with a lisp. I just could not talk. The subcontractor explained we had come to measure. He mentioned to the gentleman that I had hurt myself and couldn't talk and the gentleman thought that was my disability.

He said, "You should be helping Mr Edwards, not me today. His needs are greater than mine!"

We measured up but we didn't get the work. I think he thought I was not able to do the job properly. It taught me a lesson: never to get drunk again like that.

But again Fi was the person who picked up the pieces and I don't know how long she could have gone on like that. She had to think of what to do, because I suppose I had always been brought up surrounded by drinking and she wasn't used to that. She decided we needed to move. She wanted to get away from my past, where I could be the old Ray, a man she had never known. She met me as Ray Edwards, quad amputee, and that is the person she knows. She did not know, or I think like, Ray Edwards, builder and drinker.

So we moved from Staines to Sandhurst and bought a beautiful house. I was far enough away from the old environment of Egham to change my ways, just as Fiona hoped, and it worked. I realised I could not go drinking in Egham after work, because I then had to drive from Egham to Sandhurst. It is also too far and too expensive to get a taxi, so the drinking was put on hold, which was good. It was getting me on the road to recovery. Believe me, you need a strong person behind you. Fiona has stuck by me through thick and thin.

We were fortunate enough to have another baby called Taya. So, from those humble beginnings, starting out healthy, going through hell, I was now a dad of five children.

Living in Sandhurst, the home of the Military Academy, life began to get better.

From an early age helping my dad, I had always been a builder, so when I became a quad amputee, the question of work was paramount in my mind. What was I to do? How could I think about working without being manually busy again? I loved building, gardening, I loved anything to do with making and creating things with my hands and now they were not there.

My mind was in turmoil, trying to think of work, as a quad amputee, as a disabled person. Even today, I do not see myself as disabled; I just get on with what is to be done. I am a bionic man with odd appendages! I think in the early days you need to realise that you have to take things on step by step, and just learn to cope with it. You are not going to get everything right. It takes years and years to understand yourself and your ability to find or maybe create a job for yourself.

Now, I'm not stupid and I know that I am flexible in whatever I do, and as my dad always said, if you have good manners and you are a nice guy, and you are pretty sensible, you will get a job, whatever you do. You don't have to have massive qualifications, but as long as you are level-headed and a kind person, you can pretty much open a door and get a job somewhere. You just have to change your vocation. So I thought to myself *I have learned to use a computer in the arm-training school, I know I can do typing, I know the building trade inside out, so if I had some subcontractors working for me, I could work in an advisory and management capacity.* So that is what I set out to do. But of course the trouble was, in my mind, I still wanted to do the actual work, because no one can do it as well as I can! But I had to trust people – and I didn't trust people, I thought I knew best and that was all there was to it. My way was the only way. That's not the case in all walks of life. I had to bite my tongue, keep quiet and just accept.

I worked for the company, doing things; did a bit for Mum and Dad, did a bit for Dad's company, but it was still not me, and when Fi and I moved into our house, we had extensions done and I wanted to do them. I ended up trying to build a brick wall and made a mess of it but, as my dad always said, at least you are trying to do it. If you try to do it, you will get over the problems, and he was bloody right, bless him. I made sure that when I made mistakes, I counteracted them, so I did not make mistakes for very long. You become very clever with your artificial limbs. I wouldn't say I am an expert at everything, but if I can have a go, I will, and what I have learned is to ask for help when I need it. Especially in the workplace, don't be shy, don't be concerned that it is lowering you; asking for help is probably the best thing, it stops the frustration and basically you can get on with life a lot better. Trying to do something you can't sends you round the twist!

We are at a stage now where any disability can be overcome by listening, communicating and changing tactics. I do believe we all can do this.

We had bought this house, got married and I was stable in my mind that there was someone who was caring for me and loved me for what I am. I didn't have to fight that cause, I wasn't worried any more. In a stable relationship, any human being can fight any battle. The instability and the loneliness only cause more problems. So I think I'd got to the winning post in some ways and I was allowed to try to do things; Fi would help a bit, but she let me do my own thing. With Fiona's love, care and guidance and my dad's strength, I have been able to do most things in my life. I still truly think that is my vision, the fire in my belly. But I cannot just stand still, I have to have a purpose. So what could my purpose be? How could I use my disability to help others? How could I make this hell I had been through worthwhile?

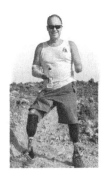

CHAPTER SIX

Out of the blue

There was a skeleton in the cupboard that one day would come out. I had told Fiona about my son Christopher, who was born on Christmas Day 1989. I didn't really get on with his mother and it was such a shame. I felt guilty I was not there for him, but circumstances had dictated the situation and I knew his mother would look after him well.

Years later, in about 2009, while working for the Limbless Association, I opened the office door one day, switched on the computer and started to read my emails, which was the first thing I did every morning. One of the emails that had come through said DO NOT THROW THIS EMAIL AWAY! PLEASE READ IT. The name was given, which I immediately recognised: it was my son Christopher.

In a nutshell it stated that he had been searching and searching to find me and pleaded with me not to delete the email. He had reasons to get in touch. He had watched me on television, he had read reports and he had searched the web to keep a track on me. He knew I was his father, but understood if I did not want to meet him, and that would be fine. He wrote: 'If you want to, I would like to meet you.' So, after reading that, feeling a bit gob-smacked and being the namby-pamby that I am, I decided I needed to ask Fiona what to do. Fiona already knew he existed, so that was not a problem. She said, "If you want to meet him, arrange it." I knew that was what I wanted to do. Fiona was behind it all the way, which was great because I am always open about things; there are no secrets between us.

But this was someone I had only seen as a baby and now he was a man aged 20. So I replied to the email, saying I would love to meet up. There was an instant reply explaining that he lived in a flat near Ham, Richmond and would love to meet me, so we arranged one Friday afternoon to meet.

It is very much like a story you read in a book, where you meet someone you haven't met for a long time, so you drive to this place and park outside the rear of the flats. I wondered what he would look like. I rang the bell and someone came down. This person was very tall, much taller than I expected. He was very good-looking, of course. We just looked at each other and I started crying.

What do you say? I eventually said, "I am so sorry."

I gave him a cuddle and words failed me for a time. He invited me in for a cold drink. How do you break the ice? What do you say? How do you have a conversation with your son for the first time when he is 20 years old? Most people at least have a build-up to the man-to-man conversation. I thought I was in for a right telling-off, because I had not been in his life. I was ready to take all the blows.

I said, "It is lovely to meet you, shall we have a chat?"

He said he would like to talk with me and so I suggested we went to the pub. I thought it would be better to be on neutral ground. It would certainly make me feel more at ease.

So we went down to the local pub and had a good chat. It was quite emotional. To think that he was my son and all these years had gone by without seeing him. It was like getting to know a stranger in many ways. But I think he was so pleased to have met his real dad. His mum has married and it is good that he has someone who is a father figure because it is important to have that. I know how close I was to my dad, it is a great feeling. I was so proud to have become part of his life again.

We had a very good chat, then went back to his flat. I said I would love to see him again and I wanted him to meet Nicola and Taya, which we arranged, and that was another emotional rollercoaster. They were meeting their half-brother, someone I didn't really know either.

I was worried how they would react, but I thought it was important for the three of them to meet. Would they understand? It was not the problem I thought it would be, but still very emotional. So, having all those thoughts in my mind, how far had I come! From being told I was unable to have children, due to the cancer, I had now met number five. Five children! I am immensely proud of all of them.

I still keep in contact with Christopher to this day. He has been to our house and he enjoys being with the family; he is a now a very successful head chef in a hotel and I just wish him all the best and send him my love. A great part of my life!

Another great part of my life was discovering one of my favourite places in the world, the place where I feel I belong: Lanzarote. Wow!

Fiona and I went to Lanzarote for the first time to stay with our friends Paul and Tina, for Paul's 50th birthday in 2003. They had a villa over there, it is beautiful. They live in a place called Costa Teguise, positioned out on the Atlantic. It is situated in a complex and the scenery and setting is idyllic.

I remember when I first landed I thought it looked like something out of the *Flintstones*, the cartoon programme: beautiful stones everywhere. I had never seen anywhere like it. That is my name for it now: Flintstones. I don't think I am Fred though!

We all went over: Fiona, Nicola, Taya who was a baby, and me. Paul is a dear friend of mine and we have all become great friends over the years. We enjoyed the 50th celebration, with plenty of swimming, laughing, drinking and having fun. It was so relaxing and enjoyable. One of the things which struck me was how kind the locals were to me. They made me feel totally at ease and for once I was able to walk around in shorts, without feeling I was different and without being stared at. They saw me as Ray, not the disabled Brit. They made me feel so welcome. The fact that I felt at ease then enabled everyone else to relax and we had a fantastic holiday.

Because of our welcome and good experiences we thought it would be wonderful to go back there again and again, somewhere where we could feel at home. We had been thinking about buying a holiday home to escape to, and Lanzarote seemed the ideal place. Paul and Tina were delighted that we would be joining them and they immediately went out to choose a property for us. They soon found one: a little bungalow with two bedrooms, which sounded just right. They told us all about it and it did seem ideal. They talked about it so positively, it seemed exactly the type of place we would like, so we went ahead to buy it. Strange really to buy a house on someone else's say-so because after all we hadn't seen it! Somehow we knew it would be fine, that everything would be OK, as we trusted Paul and Tina's judgment and it just felt so right.

So, we became the proud owners of our villa, and have been going there ever since. It is lovely to see not only Tina and Paul, but all the other friends we have made. Here we are, ten years down the line, we still have the property, but the only problem is that the flights are so expensive. However, it is a great asset to us as it enables us to chill out as a family, away from the hustle and bustle. As I have said, I don't like to be perceived as disabled, and yet once away from the UK and having my own property, there it is, home from home, and I can just be Ray. We will keep the villa forever, as a legacy for the girls, once we are no longer here. Oh wonderful place!

In my life, all of these knocks have never stopped me doing challenges.

A friend of ours at the Limbless Association said, "Why don't you meet me up at a flying school in Cranfield? Would you like to come up in a plane?"

I agreed and so he took me up in his plane. He is disabled too and loves the freedom flying gives him. We went up in the plane and it was marvellous. I could not believe it. The sights were superb and the feeling was wonderful – surreal really. I thought I would love to have a go at this. It really got my adrenalin going and the more I thought about it, the more I wanted to do it. I like to push the boundaries, to show that anyone can have a go at things, no matter how many limbs you have. So how about a quad amputee flying! It was more than I could imagine.

Anyway, in 2008 I applied to have lessons. The first lesson was the funniest. It was in a very small plane, a Cessna, and believe me, if you opened your arms wide, you could touch each door. Getting in the plane was a feat in itself. I have never been the most elegant of people and since being a quad amputee, my ability to get into and out of cars etc. has proved even more difficult. So I got in one end and out the other, because I am so awkward – I'm not delicate at all. I had to learn how to be careful: where to stand and where not to stand, for example. Much as I would have liked to, I was advised very strongly not to stand on the wing or I would put my foot through it. I didn't want to cause trouble, so I listened very carefully to my instructions.

I was thinking *I have no feeling in my feet and hands and there is this engine in front of me and I am going to be in control… this is scary.*

You have a briefing and you are literally learning in the classroom first. Then you go out in the plane and the pilot starts off. The plane taxis along the runway and you get the feel of the throttles. You have to get used to it, and using the foot pedals. You know, you are suddenly thinking *Oh my God, I can do this!*

I was very fortunate to have the first ilimb fitted to my hand. This is an electronic arm, which is a micro arm and acts on muscle impulse to control the arm. So imagine if you are opening and closing your fist, I can do so by controlling the muscles in my arm. The electronic impulse goes to my wrist to open and close the hand. I got the hand and locked it on to the yoke, which is the steering wheel of the plane.

The pilot said, "Now you will taxi along the runway, you can steer the plane by the rudders with your feet."

Remember, my feet are prosthetic. They are not like everyone else's feet. I cannot feel them, so using them for controls for the first time was a huge task. I know I drive a car, but for anyone who has ever piloted a plane, they will know the first time you are charged with controlling the plane is a very nerve-wracking ordeal. I think it is the fact of not having anything under you but air! I remember looking down, thinking *OK, so you take a left, left and then a right, right.* I had control of the throttle with my right hook. You hold on to the rudders because you brake with the rudders, unless you are braking with the pedal. So there I was, waiting, revved, ready to go. You take the foot off the brake and away you go; at 80mph, you pull the yoke back and you are there.

When the pilot has got it up so far, he says, "You are now in control!"

I am in control!

I pushed the pedals and it was absolutely awesome! I have been learning ever since. You know, I still love that feeling now. Believe me, if you can imagine, you are on a passenger flight and you are waiting for the pilot. Suddenly the co-pilot brings in a box marked 'pilot' and he puts him together, that will be me!

Whether or not they will give me a licence to carry passengers, I don't know. It would be amazing if one day a quad amputee was put on the board, I would be the first in the world.

It was terrific.

I have always had a go at things, but since being a quad amputee, once I had come to terms with it, I have had a go at anything, although that is more difficult now.

An opportunity presented itself to me in 2009. I wanted to do a skydive. Due to health conditions I was not allowed to do one, because the air at 10,000 feet is not very good. So my wife Fiona decided to do it for me with my dear friend Stan. Having had the few hours of flying, I was able to press the pilot of the Islander plane to let me get on board.

I said, "Would you mind if I took control during the flight?" He said that I needed to prove with my log book that I had enough flying hours.

So, on a very nice afternoon, we took the Islander up to 10,000 feet. Then the pilot said, "You have control," and I didn't know what to do. Everything I had learned went out of my head. I banked to the left, it went round once and then in the next second, the door was opened and the control light went green. I banked a little bit more to the left, and then out Fiona went. I had become the first quad amputee pilot to throw his wife out of a plane!

She was intact, bless her. She landed safely. Stan went out as well, but I don't think I was in control at the time and, as my wife said, it was the best experience she had ever had. It was awesome, she said. The photographs and the filming were fantastic and it was something I will never forget. Hopefully I will get back to flying. I haven't done any for a few years and I would love to get back to that, we will see.

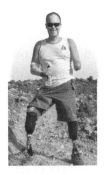

CHAPTER SEVEN

The Hardest Climb

Living in Sandhurst was, and still is, a breath of fresh air for all of us, especially Fiona. She doesn't have to cope with a drunken husband and we can live our own life, away from memories. I was now probably more at ease, but work-wise I didn't know what I wanted to do. The restless part of me was still there. I wanted to be useful. I thought about one question more and more: should I start up again in building?

But the other side of me was very interested in helping people, especially other amputees. Two years on from first becoming a quad amputee, I became a member of a charity called the Limbless Association. I thought it would be interesting to get to know and help other people who were going through the same hell, or similar. From the moment I realised what had happened to me I knew I was different, not part of the 'normal' society and I felt I needed to be part of a community. I went to their meetings. I was preparing myself for a future which I didn't know and couldn't begin to anticipate. A future that none of my close friends or family could begin to understand or know. As time went on I got quite close to the heads, the trustees. In the 1990s, I became a trustee myself. I understood the plight of amputees and what they required.

Work-wise, I went back to my father's company and helped a bit, but it was still not right. Things were not the same. I was frustrated. I felt people treated me differently, treated me as if I was wrapped in cotton wool. I believed I could do so much more.

So I formed a small company trying to adapt homes, with my knowledge of adapting my own home in Staines. What the home looked like was paramount and I understood the frustrations. When you have spent a long time in hospital and you have a disability which changes your life, you don't want a clinical home, you want an aesthetically pleasing home. I learned to cope with that in my own way, with my dad helping me. After we had finished the home in Staines, as I have mentioned we moved to Sandhurst, which had to be adapted as well. In doing so, I had become quite knowledgeable.

I really wanted to get closer to my family again. I asked my dad, who was working with my brother at that time, would he mind if I joined forces with him. I could specialise in adaptations but with Dad and Derek at the helm too. Dad thought that would be good, as he wanted to retire, so in 1998/9 we formed Edwards Brothers Ltd. We were working on adaptations, helping other people in their homes. We all worked very, very hard, going from strength to strength. We knew what to do and got on and did it. It was also good to be back in the family fold, working together again, and it was great to see Mum and Dad and everyone happy.

But like everything else, just when everything is going well, something happens. I was not prepared for what was to happen next.

It was my brother's birthday, March 22nd, I had a phone call. I was driving on the motorway, and my brother phoned me to say Dad had been rushed into hospital. He was in St Peter's Hospital in Chertsey. He had an aneurism and was seriously ill. I was shocked, I didn't know what to do. Dad couldn't be ill, he had always been there for me. He was the voice of reason. He kept my metaphorical feet on the ground.

I don't remember much about what happened next. I went to the hospital, Mum was there with Derek and time seemed to stand still. We just sat and waited – waited for Dad to recover but unfortunately that was not to be so. Dad passed away that day, on my brother's birthday. It was quite poignant that day really considering what had happened on Dad's birthday before, but this time it wasn't something that happened to me. It was such a big shock. Dad had affected so much of my life and I loved him so much; I didn't know what I was going to do. My mentor had passed away, my rock. We sat as a family and did what most families do: grieve in our own way. We thought of

Dad in our happy days. Well, we lived to cope with those things but I know he will never, ever be out of my mind. I do feel sad that my second daughter Taya did not get to meet her granddad. I think he is my angel as well and he is still with me today.

I feel that losing our dad, my brother and I coped with it in different ways. Derek coped with it by going to clubs and trying to forget, which we can all understand in some ways.

Unfortunately, things got a bit upsetting for my brother and his family. Maybe too much entertainment. Things were not good for Derek and his wife in the marital home. They were not happy and so there was going to be a parting of the ways. It didn't help running the business at this time, there was more and more pressure. What had started out so well was just not working. I don't know if it was not having Dad around or whether Derek and I were just not in a good place. Eventually, after a lot of soul searching on my part, in 2003 we had to dissolve that company. It was very sad.

But what was I to do now, where had my whole working life gone? I was still a trustee of the Limbless Association and I was very much involved in trying to get our charity right, along with the other trustees. I wanted to do things for other people. So, a few months on from when the company was dissolved, I formed Access UK Ltd. All my experience and knowledge in the construction industry and adaptation business brought this company to quite a strong position, adapting homes in the South-East, working with colleagues I used to know.

But unfortunately in those days, I was a very hands-on director. That was the only way I knew. This is really difficult when you are disabled, especially when you do not have the dexterity in your hands. I felt very frustrated when I went on site, knowing that I could have once done a better job. Unfortunately, when you rely on other people, we all know they let us down sometimes. I think the frustration of employing subcontractors was a whole nightmare. This, combined with losing Dad and all the pressure, meant I was bound to be heading for a misfortune again. I felt there had to be something about to happen. I only wish I had not been right!

In July 2005, Fiona and I left to go on a long-needed holiday in Lanzarote. On 27th July, while still on holiday, I had a phone call from the UK. It was my niece, telling me my brother had died. Believe me, when you are sitting round the swimming pool and you get that phone call you are just shocked. You are numb. My brother being eight years younger, I thought *Oh my God…* I thought of my mum, because my dad wasn't there, so what should I do? I told Fiona and she said that I must get back to my mum, so we booked a flight. But prior to that, I went to the bar by the swimming pool and had a few shots to calm me down.

I flew back to the UK two days later. Unfortunately, Derek died in Thailand, so my nieces went there and brought the body back and we buried him in Englefield Green near my dad in St Jude's church, where I went to Sunday school. The family thing really. We had buried my dad, now my brother, and for my mum to bury her son was not nice at all. We were all very tearful, very sad. He was at rest now. Sad for his children. I hope they think of the good times rather than the bad.

Again, we got over that trauma, but oh my God, what more is going to hit this family? When we all got back, we got on with our lives, as it were, still thinking about our loved ones.

In October, Fiona and I were due to go out to Lanzarote again with the family, for a break. Our flight was on a Thursday. On the Tuesday, very early, I woke up with severe chest pains.

I said, "There is something wrong here."

Fiona thought I had man-flu, a cold or something. But it felt like I had an elephant sitting on my chest. So we called the NHS helpline. I spoke to someone, and I know the question was: "How are you?" and I told them I was not feeling well and I was breathing a bit unhealthily, struggling for breath. I was not feeling well at all. I got up to go to the bathroom and collapsed for a couple of seconds. I bit my tongue when I fell. Eventually an ambulance was called and I was given an aspirin under my tongue and I ended up in Frimley Park Hospital. That was quite traumatic because I asked the consultant looking after me what was the matter and he told me I was having a heart attack.

Thank you very much! was all I could think.

Having no arms, the drip had to be put in my neck, and I remember being asked if I had cut myself. The reason why I was asked is that wherever I had a cut would swell up. I had forgotten my fall in the bathroom, my bitten tongue, and so I said no.

You can imagine: this liquid was being pumped into me so my mouth swelled up. I couldn't talk, and I talk so much – this was my pay-back I think. When you can't talk properly and you are being asked questions, it is very difficult. I had been terribly ill and I was just out of it. They gave me X-rays and tests and told me how poorly I was.

It is funny the things that go through your mind when you are ill. You would think with all I had been through I would know about being out of it with drugs and the strange things you ask, but no. All I could think about was getting out of there and going on my holiday. I thought that would be the thing to make me feel better. I managed to speak to ask if I would be better for Thursday when we were flying to Lanzarote for a week.

The consultant said, "Mr Edwards, you will be lucky if you could go to the moon, the way you are going. You are very seriously ill."

Unfortunately they found there was a litre and a half of fluid around my heart and damage to the left-hand side, so I was in a state.

So, one day in intensive care and a further six days in hospital and then seven days at Atkinson Morley, having invasive surgery, like an angiogram: tube up the groin and then linked into the heart. I am now not only bionic outside but also bionic inside! This was the most frightening part of my life, where I was thinking that I was never leaving this mortal coil. I had fought so many battles, but now my engine room was not working properly. I know it seems funny, but the arms and legs and the cancer I could cope with, but the heart was something different. It was very hard to cope with a difficulty there. What do you do after that? What do you think to yourself? Do you take stock? But I had taken stock since 1981, I didn't know what else I could do. Believe me, I said to myself, I cannot and will not go through any more. This is the limit. How much does a human being have to take? One thing I knew, if I survived this, I could survive anything. Thinking about our troops coming back, I can empathise with everything they go through. I had been through three war zones!

Two weeks went by and I slowly recovered. Again, I couldn't wait to get home to recuperate. I had had enough of hospitals for a lifetime.

Well, two or three weeks went by at home before I was allowed to drive and get back on with my life. Touch wood, things have been pretty good.

The only thing is, the company I had, Access UK Ltd, was still ticking over, but I had to call it a day because I couldn't cope with people letting me down. I couldn't take the stress. So I just closed the company, continuing to be a trustee for the Limbless Association and in my own way. I said I thought I should run the charity, because they were a bit haphazard, and so they asked me to come on board and gave me the job of deputy chief executive officer. That was the first time I had been involved with charity work and it opened my eyes to see how charities are so much like business. So much paperwork, so much bureaucracy! People are so jealous of each other.

That was in 2006; I managed to get over that and gradually took up the role of acting chief executive officer.

While I was there I always wanted to do fund-raising and that type of thing. I did bikeathons and went around the country talking at many of the centres, trying to promote, help and assist amputees and their families. Making them aware that life is still OK. As an amputee, who better than me to be in a position to do that?

In 2009, on a nice summer's day at home, we decided to have a barbeque. Barbeque parties are just our thing. My wife and I invited loads of friends. We were in our hot tub with a few friends, chatting away, red wine was flowing, and we were all certainly quite merry by then.

My dear friend Stan said, "Ray, why don't you go for a walk?"

I said, "Don't be stupid, I am sitting in a hot tub."

"No, why don't you do an expedition, do a challenge?"

"Like what?"

"Let's climb Kilimanjaro."

So in my drunken, stupid state I said, "Yes, I will do anything."

Next morning, with a bit of a headache, I told my wife what I had done and she then looked on the internet to see what I had agreed to do. When I found out Kilimanjaro was 5200 metres, that means altitude, and I have had a heart attack. What a silly situation to be in!

I still said OK, I am a man of my word, so we set ourselves the task of getting a team together.

We arranged to meet up, all of us, to begin training. It took a lot of training. We went to Dartmoor and Ben Nevis. The biggest challenge you could face, other than learning about how to deal with the altitude, because that was something we had to deal with, and nothing is going to compare with Kilimanjaro, was that I needed the sheer stamina. Would the body take it? Would the stumps take it because the consideration was not only me, but would the components of the limbs take it? There was one quad amputee – myself – and a gentleman called Mark. He had amputation above the knee and he had osteo-integration, which is a pin coming out of the bone. He had like a skeleton structure which was working on a knee joint which was powered by electrics. The only way to achieve this was with a power pack on his back. We called him Battery Boy. There were two other guys who had lost a limb below the knee.

So in 2010, 24 people, including Stan and me, went to Kilimanjaro, four of whom were amputees.

We flew to Nairobi, and then flew on towards Kili. We thought Kili would be dead and deserted, but it wasn't. It was like an international airport. There were people all around and they were lovely. We went straight to the Kia Lodge; awesome these lodges, there were swimming pools and all that, such luxury. Yet you could see in the distance this pimple and the pimple was Kilimanjaro. It was a big pimple! In the foreground you could see elephants and giraffes; it was beautiful, an idyllic setting.

The next day, prior to going up to Kili, we went to the medical centre just outside Kilimanjaro, called the Moshi medical centre. I met with the dean, Harold Shengarli. Harold showed all the team how they set up their limb centre and how they helped people who had lost their limbs. I didn't realise it cost $500 to buy an artificial leg. Where would the amputees there get that amount of money? Most of them did not know where the next meal was coming from. It dawned on me, talking to them, that we could try to help them. We could get things made. I thought if I could do something for them, I would. They appreciated this and said anything would help them. But at the moment the thing on my mind was beginning to climb this beautiful mountain.

With this Kilimanjaro climb, I suppose I was very blasé about it; I took it on the chin and didn't realise what I personally had set myself to do. I mean, I had never even camped in a tent as a quad amputee, I didn't know what the bloody hell I was doing. We were all a team; we were just following each other, doing a bit of walking and training. Everyday work was getting up, going to work and then you do this! It only dawned on me what I had agreed to when I camped out a few times during the training and I found it a bit difficult, but I still muddled through. But was I really ready in my mind to do this Kilimanjaro challenge? Would I ever have been ready? I think the answer is no. I blinkered myself thinking *I'll just go with the flow* and even on the plane going over from the UK, landing at Kili, there was an elation just landing there, but deep down I was thinking *Oh dear!* I didn't want to admit it, even to myself.

I know my fellow climbers, in particular certain people who were there to help in my domestic duties, would look out for me. They had volunteered and they were lovely: Laura, Maggie and Lisa. They are caring people because they are from the health industry, but was I really ready mentally?

It was a tough challenge from day one: the dust, the trauma, the crying. It was 20 degrees in the daytime and -15 degrees at night. As a quad amputee, it is very tough living in a tent. I can remember one evening when I had my arse hanging out of the tent; I was trying to get in, to get warm, everywhere was dark and this was in no way camping in a luxury way. This was one of the hardest things I had ever done in my life, mainly because I was doing it on my own. No one could tell me what it was like as a quad amputee. I was trail blazing again.

The first day we arrived at the camp late, after a horrible walk. I thought *Why the hell am I trundling up a sodding mountain? I have never wanted to or enjoyed doing this sort of thing in my life!* Then I had a reality check as to why I was there: to give a bit of hope to people of what they can do with a disability. You know, it dawned on me: this is bloody horrible, I am lifting my legs over rocks and people are trying to help me to do it. Yeah, we are singing songs; yes, there is a rally cry; and yeah, as one human being to another human being we are having fun. But then we get to put up the tents and I am thinking what I have to do. I have got my rucksack. The tent is up and my bed's laid out, but I know I have got to strip off and I can't do zips properly, I can't do buttons and this is only day one! How the hell am I going to do it? I hated having to rely on people. Fiona and Mum are not here, the people I am comfortable with caring for me. I am going into baby stage thinking *What am I going to do?*

That night, we just slept and you get woken up in the morning with a cup of tea made for you and they were all happy, but I was as miserable as sin. I am always a bit grumpy in the morning. We ate breakfast, but someone had to help me to do this; in an environment like that it's your tent fellow, in my case this was Albert. He was brilliant, but I had to wait for my carers to help me. They were very kind, but it was not good for me mentally. You feel as though you are not in control; you are not independent. This is what dawned on me and we were many, many miles away from the cotton wool world of home and my lovely bed and my lovely family. All I had was a small tent, where I hit my head when I tried to stand up, and my arse was outside the tent door when I lay down, or moved. It was just bloody stupid!

Naturally, we all have to go to the toilet and when the tents are laid out and you get up after your day's gruelling trip, walking and clambering over rocks, you get in your tent after dinner and there is always a time when the bodily functions work. By then, frost is on the ground and it is bloody cold. Added to this, I hadn't got my legs on, and I wanted to go to the toilet, and I mean really wanted to go. Earlier in the evening you have a washbowl, in order to have a wash. The bowl is put outside. I thought *I can't crawl across the rocks to the toilet.* My tent mate was fast asleep so I opened the inner liner of the tent and there was the bowl in the outer part of the tent. So I am afraid I had to dump in the bowl. The thing is, it had ice all the way round the rim and it stuck to my arse. So I was stuck in this bowl, halfway out of the tent, in the outside part of the tent. It was freezing cold. Eventually the heat of my body melted the ice and I had finished my duty and I slipped the bowl outside the tent. The next morning everyone on the site was talking about the fact that an animal must have been around the camp during the night because of what it had left. The rumour was it was a wolf! Unfortunately, I had to own up. That was one of the very embarrassing moments I had. Believe me, even the toilet tent itself was just a wooden seat with a bucket and many times I sat on it and fell off. It was absolute hell on earth. It was certainly not five-star accommodation and terrible for a quad amputee.

The porters got to know me early on, thinking *Why? It's Raymondo comma Simba: Raymondo the lion. This is mad! We don't send people up mountains with no arms or legs! If we do, we send them a different way.* I was going the Lemosho route and there is Coca-Cola route which is easier. Well, thanks for telling me!

You think to yourself *Let's plod on* and the lead guy tells you what to do, but it went in one ear and out the other. It was like I was on a conveyor belt, I just got up and went. Roy Valentine, who I must say was my hero, was my neighbour and my mate. He just said, "Come on mate," and we became great friends. I was just following him really. We helped each other but actually I couldn't understand why I was doing it. At the end of the day, I just wanted it to end. There was great comradeship, having meals and fun, but the routine of trundling over rocks and the dust was an experience and I suppose it was all right, but I was frightened of not being in control. That was the problem. I think I cried a lot to myself. I was upset, but I didn't show it much because I know how to put on a brave face, but I suppose the challenges in my life have made me not like to be out of control. I have to see an ending and I just wanted to beat it; I just wanted to say I had achieved the climb as a disabled person. I never wanted to do it when I was able-bodied!

Getting into day two, day three, day four, it is still tough, it doesn't get any easier. You see little mountains you have to climb and you think *What the bloody hell am I doing?* I had to wait for my carers to help and they were brilliant. They used to hold my rucksack, because it was too heavy for me to manage. On the second day it rained and that was when I got a chill. This developed into a chest infection, and I was put on antibiotics. The people who were experienced were telling me I couldn't do this, I couldn't carry on. The higher you go, the less oxygen you have and I was struggling for breath. You see people on these challenges, and these expeditions are not a walk in the park; I take my hat off to anybody who takes on these challenges.

And of course, there are times when you have walked and walked, especially on artificial limbs, like you do on your feet, you get blisters. Well, the residual limbs, the stumps, were suffering with blisters. There is this Compeed, which is like plasters, you can put on to stop or help the blisters. After day three, each of my limbs had about six or seven Compeeds on them. It was hell, the rubbing. I think that was the worst part of the walk. You are putting your limb through something it is not expected to do. The makers of the limbs don't design them to do these challenges. They are to be used to live life normally, as you can. Just normal walking. When I got back to the UK with all these Compeeds on my limbs, it took days and days to take them off. You can't just rip them off, like you do plasters. You have to soak them. If you rip them off, half your skin comes with it. That was hell on earth, believe me. It took a long time for me to recover, physically and mentally. I must say, I appreciate home cooking, home life, everything about home much more now.

Some of the team had coughs and colds, due to altitude and tiredness. But, as I said, team spirit was essential. We had medical advice, we had doctors, and we had a good team leader. But it was probably day six when they found out I was seriously ill with a chest infection. Having no spleen and having had a heart attack within the last five years, they were not too sure that I was going to make it.

I was so poorly that night, they said, "Ray, you can't go on any more."

"Why?"

"You just can't."

They sat me in the tent and gave me a cup of tea, and they brought in this bag. I asked them what the bag was for and they replied that it was a body bag. I asked them why they had brought the bag into the tent. They answered that if I went any further, I wouldn't be coming back walking, I would be coming back in the body bag. So, they made my decision for me: I could not go on. I was very tearful.

The next morning I knew they were continuing up, to finish the job, and I ended up being sung to by the whole team. It was very emotional. They brought me down on a stretcher. It was hell on earth. There was another guy

who was brought down with me. I just wanted to do it…
I take full account of what I did and I thank all the people
who helped me do it. Ronaldo, my guide, was helpful as
well, and my team mates. But it ended up with me being
ill, I couldn't speak, I was vomiting. I was quite pleased at
the end of the day that I was back down, because it was
just hell. I was very upset in my own thoughts and I would
have been so proud to stand on the summit and say I had
done it.

When I got a bit better, nowhere near as poorly, we
walked up to see the remainder of the team coming
down; they had completed the challenge. They had
reached the summit: 17 out of 24. We were elated. We
were in a little village and everyone was pleased. Some
way, however poor they are, it does not stop them being
kind. The Tanzanian people are lovely. Sweets are like
huge wealth to them: you have won the lottery, here is a
bag of sweets.

I remember I spied in the distance, in the village, two
amputees. One was about 11 years old and the other
about 13. He also had one arm missing. Well, they had
never seen anyone with artificial arms and legs and I
thought *Oh my God!*

I had already heard that one of the boys had his arm
removed through an argument with his stepmother, who
sliced his arm off. How wicked was that? The other one
had cancer. I thought about the experience I had on that
mountain: like all experiences, you could not buy this.

When you have a disability and you have a problem medically, you really should listen to what other people say. I was told it was best to sit at a desk and watch other people do things. But that is not me, who has got no brain sometimes. People have said: "Ray, to get to where you did is an achievement on its own." I think to have suffered the humiliation and not being independent taught me a massive lesson. I know from these experiences of the cold, which was -15 at night to 25 degrees in the day, the views will never go away and they were awesome, but I personally would never want to put my body through that again. It was hell, but the experience was fantastic!

When we arrived back at Heathrow, we were very pleased to be on British territory. The actual trip and the challenge were enormous. We had raised £86,000 for the amputee community. Unfortunately, I was made redundant, so had another challenge to come.

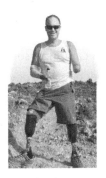

CHAPTER EIGHT

Another birth: Limbcare

Looking back on my life, I realise now that the experiences I have been through have taught me a lot of lessons and changed me as a person. They have given me a lot more patience, understanding and so much knowledge to give out to other people. Would it have happened otherwise? No one knows, but I am sure that when you have a few knocks and it then turns your life around, it makes you take stock and think about things more carefully. It makes you analyse human nature and think about what is important to you and then consider others.

Before all this, would I have ever even thought about running a charity? I don't think so. I truly believe your destiny is set out for you in life and, when it came to it, Limbcare was a vision that happened in 1987, while lying in hospital, and came to fruition in 2010. Along that road, I have been a builder, a husband twice, a family man. In the back of my mind, whatever was happening, I have always been a caring person, but that side of me never came out, never began to develop until I became a quad amputee. I was in a challenging position and it was through that I thought about the help and support I got and needed, which made me think about how I could help and support others in a similar position. I had to begin life all over again really: learning to walk, learning to use my arms and legs. I have tried my best to get over my disability in a positive way and with Fiona's help and the support of my family, I have created quite a good life. Yes, I have bad days, everyone does, but Limbcare is my baby – it was meant to be!

I had worked for a charity and had been a builder, so armed with all that knowledge, and knowing full well that I couldn't get to the summit of that bloody volcano called Kilimanjaro, then made redundant, what was I to do?

Limbcare was the saving grace. It was the reason I had gone through everything. It was my goal for the future, my purpose in life. So how did I form Limbcare? Well, I happened to know two amputees and a good colleague of mine I worked with; there was Alex, my deputy CEO, and Barry and Roy, both amputees. The four of us, under my guidance, decided to form Limbcare: a charity giving hope, support and help to amputees and their families, to enable them to have a better quality of life. This was a big challenge because any charity is like forming a company, but I knew in my heart of hearts I was doing the right thing. Never in my wildest dreams did I think it would be so tough, but being the type of person I am, including a good communicator, I got people to rally round and sponsor certain things for us. So Limbcare became a charity on June 8th 2010. What a great achievement. To start with, we had to work from home, we had no finance, but all I wanted to do was help people. We had no help-line, no support, all I had was my mobile.

I still had contact with Roehampton Hospital, as I still attended it from time to time, so I spoke to the manager to ask if we could have a support desk there. They agreed to this, which was great. I had got over one hurdle, as I could now offer a service of support, a support desk, under the Limbcare banner. I was so proud, because this was the hospital that rebuilt me and now I was giving something back. What a great feeling that is and you saw the new amputees coming in and we could offer support. I knew it would help, because I know that when I was in that situation I wish I had had a quad amputee to talk to me and help me with all the challenges and frustrations I faced. Using my strength of character, along with my colleagues, we were helping others.

We went from strength to strength. We went to the other centres and spoke to all the people concerned who run the centres – all 43 of them! Gradually, over the years since we started, Limbcare has created a unique body of people, now called ambassadors – all amputees who have the same devotion and insight into helping others. It is rather like pyramid selling: the team at the top, me as chairman, and all my team, my flock, giving help and support. It is growing and growing.

In October 2010 I had a call from the cabinet office. It stated that the Queen was honouring me with the MBE. It would seem it was the work I had done for the amputees community since 2007. That meant it was a few years prior to me starting my own charity.

So, in the New Year's honours list in 2011, I became a Member of the British Empire. Wow, how about that!

I think, no I know, my dad would have been so proud. What a great thing to have bestowed on you. I was proud as a peacock. Absolutely! So was my family.

We found out that the ceremony was to be held on 6th May 2011 at Windsor Castle. Her Majesty would be there to bestow the honour on me.

It is a costly affair. My wife and girls wanted new dresses and I had to rent a tail suit. You are really dressed up to the nines. The car was polished and we had a friend of mine chauffeur it for us.

When you go to Windsor Castle, drive down The Long Walk. The sun was shining and, as I am a disabled person, we had a special badge pass to take us through to the castle. Oh Wow! Not many people have the pleasure of driving their car through those gates. You arrive and the policemen on duty open the car doors, and escort you to the castle itself.

We went up a beautiful staircase lined with soldiers and officers. My wife and my girls were invited to withdraw into another room, to be looked after until they went into the audience to watch the procedure. I was taken into a lovely room where all the awards are bestowed: MBE's OBE's and Knighthoods.

I was given a glass of wine, it was beautiful!

A lot of people were called up and went in groups. We were the third group to go in. We followed the officer in charge who took us towards the room where Her Majesty was. Music was playing on the balcony; the audience of all the families was there and soldiers, officers and dignitaries. It was so posh and typically British. As I got nearer to the opening I suddenly saw Her Majesty in view. Oh my gosh - it certainly is a wow factor! I was second in line to be called up to Her Majesty and told quietly by one of the officers standing by, "Do not move until you hear your name." There were butterflies in my stomach.

Suddenly I heard, "Ray Edwards MBE, on behalf of the amputee community in the United Kingdom, for his charitable work."

I went up and bowed in front of Her Majesty as she walked forward. She would normally take your hand, but in my case it was my artificial hook. She said in her beautiful voice, "I have read about you. You have done so much for the amputee community. May I ask, how did you lose your arm?"

"Ma'am, I have lost my four limbs."

"Well done."

I think it wasn't so much a faux pas, but more a well done for all I had gone through. She asked me more questions about my life and I explained I run a charity looking after human beings and I just wanted to help people. She seemed to understand and be so pleased. I am sure she speaks to so many people, as we all know, but in those particular few seconds, or minutes, I was talking to her and it was my moment. She asked me what I was doing afterwards and luckily Fiona had set up a wonderful party at Runnymede Hotel, so I told her.

"Oh lovely," she said, "I do hope you enjoy it."

So we had photographs taken and then got back in the car and drove to Runnymede to enjoy our lovely afternoon. It was a day I will never forget, thanks to Fiona.

A beautiful, beautiful day!

We have been lucky enough to be on television and in the summer of 2013 we were interviewed on *The One Show* on BBC One, but our biggest gift is that we visit people in hospitals. I only know that if you are an amputee and you see another amputee walking towards you, it does give you a lot of hope: knowing there is a future to look at, rather than seeing a blank wall. Yes, people are going to get frustrated; yes, there are so many questions, we have them from the families as well, but if we can offer support and help in the UK, I am very proud to have done my job. For me personally, my journey has been another huge challenge with Limbcare.

The support and help we give is in many, many ways, but I suppose the most important thing is to help with benefit advice, talk to the young amputees to tell them the road to recovery is OK. We try to guide them into the right frame of mind, offer support when they need it, but tell them if they have any problems at all (such as fitting of the limb, the centre or any problems at home, including arguing) we can advise by way of offering them professional consultation. We are not going to be able to do everything and we don't try, but we have the back-up of many professionals who can help us. When you contact us by phone, there is an instant response from a person at the other end, especially now we have a support line 24/7. The best person to talk to is another amputee. It is all very well having a call centre, but I truly believe, from my experience, we all want to talk to someone who has been through it a bit. Having been through the loss of all four limbs, and other medical traumas, I don't think you can get anyone better than me! I have people phoning up saying how they have lost a leg and my reply at times is, "Well, you are lucky really, because I have lost all four limbs!" It is not what they want to hear; yes, it is bereavement and yes, it is a very traumatic situation, but the old story is there is always someone worse off than you and life can still be worth living. Having someone at the end of a phone helps.

There is a saying: 'A problem shared is a problem halved' and we are always good listeners. That is the main criterion for Limbcare: to be a good listener. We have a lot of visits to the hospitals and, of course, Queen Mary's in Roehampton is my Mecca; I call it my Lourdes, where I go and pray that thank God they rebuilt me. I am often up there and we are very lucky to have a support desk, and we now have ambassadors all around the country, from Carlisle down to Plymouth, across to Kent and in the West Country.

One day I was in Roehampton and I met with a gentleman called John. He was a builder and Oh my God, déjà vu! He had become a quad amputee; his story is very similar to mine. Maybe this is why I am meant to be doing what I am doing. I saw him a few months ago in a wheelchair and it was like looking at me, all those years ago.

How proud and emotional I was to go up to him and say, "Hi, I'm Ray and oh my gosh, it is like looking at myself."

I have spoken to him many times since; only the other day I sat with him on the bed where he is being rehabilitated and I can honestly say, from my heart, I know exactly the journey he is on. I know exactly where he is, every day, and I told him I will be there for him. He has gone through a six-week course of learning how to put his arms and legs on.

While he was doing this he said, "I can't even wipe my bottom properly!"

I said, "I know John, it is hell!"

"I don't know what to do," he replied.

I have given him some advice and he talks to me about things; I have also spoken with his wife, Rose. They live in Southampton, so it is quite a journey for his wife to visit him in Roehampton. I have told her not to worry, as I am there for him as well and she is so pleased he has someone to depend on, to help him. I gave him an ultimatum that he would walk out of hospital and two weeks later he would be at our Gala Dinner. He was determined to be there, and he was. It was the best gift this year to see him achieve that. What an accolade for both of us, both quad amputees. Builders, to have a good old cuddle, a men's cuddle! He cried the other day and thanked me for my support and I think it sums it up what Limbcare is all about. I will be there for him all his life, as I would for anyone. I just know this is my life; this is what it is all about. I am so honoured to be able to help these people, along with my team. That is it now: I am only as good as the team. I think I have created something wonderful which will grow and grow. We are the unsexy side of the amputee community; we are not soldiers, but we have been through wars in different ways.

In the recent years of military conflict, our soldiers are coming back injured and many of them have lost limbs. I always maintain they have been such a force and helped the limb community profile to the public. They come back, get the limbs and it doesn't look like a leg now, they have proper modular limbs and they are powerful. I remember sitting with a soldier who had lost three limbs. He was devastated. He was living in a flat on the sixth floor. We helped him try to get out of there, along with the army charities, and he is now in a bungalow on his own. Civilians also need our help. There is also a future goal for Limbcare. I am very lucky to have met with Bryn Parry and his team from Help for Heroes. Living in Sandhurst I meet with the soldiers and Limbcare is now part of the hub to help the injured soldiers integrate into society and become civilians. It is very tough for an injured soldier to go through the trauma of not only losing a limb, but also then being forced into a different type of life. We are there on the civilian side. We are very closely linked with the Personal Recovery Unit (PRU) in Aldershot. We are often there as part of the charities. We are a civilian charity, but that does not matter, we are all the same. I can remember and know to this day, on certain times when we are collecting at supermarkets, 95% of people assume we are ex-service people.

They ask: "Where were you? Afghanistan or Iraq?"

That is the perception, but we don't mind because it is a talking point.

If we could only be 25% as strong as Help for Heroes, I as chairman would be so proud that when the soldiers finish their duty, we are there to support them.

I know personally that I have met so many incredible people, it has been an honour: young ladies, children. I met a young lady who is only five years old and she is a quad amputee, and can you imagine the feeling I had sitting with her? It was not her who needed help, it was her mum and dad. The families need help more at times than the person themselves. I was in the office when I took a call from her mum and dad, Jenny and Alex. Their daughter is called Charlotte. I was told she is a quad amputee, due to meningitis. She became a quad amputee in 2010. I thought *Wow! She is like me.* The parents needed more help than the child, to understand how she is going to overcome the minefield of problems and how she is going to cope.

I was invited to their home in Oxford and on the way there I thought about how I would approach talking to this five-year-old child about what things were like. What hope could I give her? What could I say to such a lovely little girl who has had such a trauma? Really it was the parents who had been through the trauma more than the little girl.

I knocked at the door and when it opened I could see Charlotte inside, without her limbs on. She was walking on her knees and she was a bit shy. She didn't come into the lounge to meet me, but I saw her pink legs lying there against the sofa. I was in a suit, so she didn't realise I am a quad amputee and I said hello, but she was still unsure. I rolled my trousers up, so she could see the artificial legs. I showed her my artificial arms: one is a carbon gripper and the other just looks like a hand. I think she was surprised.

I said, "I am just like you."

She said, "No you're not, you're a man."

So we did start to play and talk and I thought she was a cheeky little madam, but very sweet.

I saw her pink legs and said, "I like your legs, do you think I could have some like them?"

"Don't be silly, boys don't wear pink!" she said.

"Well, I would and I would like a pair like that. Will you try them on to show me what they look like please?"

She put them on and I don't know what it was, but there was a bond immediately and I thought *I am going to help you.*

It helped her parents to know there are people out there who do not see Charlotte as different and want to help her have as normal a life as possible. I knew I would help her. I know I am not a young man and certainly not a female, but I have been through a lot of what she is going through and will go through.

After many visits, Jenny, Charlotte's mum, is now the patron of Limbcare and Charlotte is the face of Limbcare Youth. It is so lovely to have her as our figurehead and with the hedgehogs, or Prickle Power team: they are the little cuddly models that show us how we as human beings, under the guise of hedgehogs, experience so many different things, and can support each other in so many aspects.

I hope, from now onwards, that I, in the form of Limbcare Youth, can develop a new path, a new beginning for the voice of Limbcare Youth.

They are our ambassadors, they are our future and nothing is cotton woolled anymore. We are there as human beings. Meningitis is on the increase, people are going through that all the time.

All I want to create is a united amputee world, a family. Many people lose limbs through diabetes; we need to look at the quality of life, healthy eating, healthy mind, healthy body. We need to look after the youth of this world. We also need to make a better world for an amputee with the fitting of the limbs: education, training for prosthetists and technicians and become a charity helping amputees in the UK. Limbcare is there for everybody, and all my team are very professional. While I have got breath in my body I will assure everyone in this country that I will be there with my team.

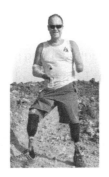

CHAPTER NINE

Raising the Profile

As a matter of course, my life turns around every day to something new. In late September/early October 2013 I had a call from my friend Reuben. He is an amputee and does a bit of filming with the Army.

He said, "Ray, how are you?"

I said, "Fine, happy day as usual."

"Done any filming?"

I answered no.

"I'm on a film set and the casting director is looking for a man with no arms."

"That's difficult, isn't it? Where are you going to find one of them?"

I was surprised when the reply was, "No, you, you idiot. Would you like to do it?"

He said he didn't know what it was really all about, but he knew it was something like a *Law and Order* type of programme and did I want my name put forward. I agreed, but then thought nothing more of it. I have never acted in my life, apart from the fool. You can imagine the surprise when I got a call from Kudos, a film company. A gentleman called Matt spoke to me, introducing himself as the second director of *Law and Order UK*. I thought about it for a moment and realised it was the programme on ITV with Bradley Walsh in it.

Matt had seen my website, seen my charity and he said, "What do you think about it? Do you fancy doing a bit of acting?"

"Is it a speaking part?" I was a bit apprehensive about that, as I didn't know if I would be able to remember lines.

"No, you are a dead body!"

I thought *Oh my gosh*. Now I see the funny side of everything, so I thought *That's another feather in my cap*! They asked me if I would do it, so I thought *In for a penny, in for a pound*. I told them I didn't have any legs either, because I know that sometimes this causes problems, especially if they wanted me to do some particular things. But they said that would not be a problem, so I said yes.

It was only after this, a little while later, I thought *If I am a dead body, what are they going to do?*

Time went on a bit and then I got another phone call, explaining that my character was a Jewish jeweller called Harry. This Harry Bernstein, the jeweller, had been in a bit of a conflict and knew a bit about a gang. The gang find him and hit him on the head, which kills him. I think he had been in various situations, but they need to remove his identity, so they cut his arms off. As you can see, this is where I came in. They take his teeth out too.

Well, I do still have some teeth and I thought *This is going a bit too far*, so I said to the producer, "Look, I will do anything, but I do want to keep a few of my teeth!"

Anyway, my age group was right, so I got the part.

On the first day of filming a car picked me up. It really was like being an actor now. I was taken to a prosthetic studio in Slough, where a cast of my upper limbs was taken so they could make my stumps look as if my arms had just been cut off. The arms looked so realistic, with the bones showing through. They cast that and I had a good chat and met the people. It really is amazing what these people make for television programmes and films.

On Wednesday 13th November I was picked up by a car and taken to Longcross studios, near Chertsey. I couldn't believe I was going to a film studio. The part I was filming was the morgue scene. What a first experience of filming. What a way to begin an acting career!

I got dropped off and there were lots of caravans everywhere, all with signs saying who they belonged to: film crew, make-up etc. Matt, the producer, introduced himself again and introduced me to a couple of people and then told me he would take me to my caravan. I was taken to this caravan, like a mobile home, and on the door it said 'Harry'. I thought *Who the hell is Harry? Who am I sharing with?* Of course, Harry was me, my character, my stage name! Fancy having your own caravan! I could see the funny side of it. I went in and there were chairs and a table and on the table was a tray of drinks. Well, that would be lovely, but my worry was that I dared not drink too much because without my artificial limbs it is really difficult for me to go to the toilet. So I couldn't really enjoy the hospitality and refreshments they were giving me.

I waited about 20 minutes before I was called to make-up. The make-up is very visual and I thought *If I am a body and they are doing the autopsy, what will they do to me?* They made me look like I had a scar, a Y-section scar on my neck which looked so realistic. They made my face look black and blue, to appear it had been bruised. They then put the prosthetic parts on my arms, my stumps. The way they made the parts, with the blood etc., it looked so realistic, like it had just happened. I was then taken in another car to the area where I was going to be filmed: in my case, this was the morgue. I went through a few pre-runs, to know what I was doing, and as I was lying out on the slab it was very difficult to hold my breath. With Bradley Walsh being a bit of a comedian as well, he and I had some jokes. We have the same sense of humour.

He said, "Come on Ray, stop making me laugh." And I said the same to him.

Although it was only 60 seconds to hold my breath, oh my God, it was so difficult to do, to concentrate. The way I did this was to listen to them doing their lines and in the end I knew their lines better than they did.

So two and a half hours in make-up and about two and a half hours of filming for a maximum of one minute of film. But the most interesting part was to meet the people and see how many people there are on the set for such a small amount of broadcast. It took another hour to remove the make-up. Of course, I still had the car crash scene. My wife and daughters were allowed to come to this part of the filming, which was brilliant. We all got to experience what it is like on a film set and had a snapshot of what an actor's life is like. Not all glamour and glitz I can tell you when you are lying on the cold floor, in the rain, pretending to be dead! But at least now I can say I am an actor.

When you become a person who is odd, like myself, the press sometimes pick up on that: quad amputee, trying to climb mountains, trying to fly planes, trying to be the village idiot really. You're beginning to put your head above the parapet; you are becoming more than a normal human being, if there is such a thing. I think media and the press love it. When I climbed Kilimanjaro, or tried to, we visited a centre and wanted to help so much. I saw people who have nothing and it made me want to do something to help them. Some had lost limbs, but they did not have the luxury of prosthetic limbs like I have. I wanted to help them, as I knew a little part of what they would be suffering. I said I would try to help. When I came back to the UK and formed Limbcare, I thought about how we could help them. I remember being in a centre where they fit the limbs and I saw there was a lot of wastage. Limbs are thrown away: either someone has passed away and the limbs are not useable, or it can be that the limb doesn't fit any more. Due to health and safety, which is an absolute mockery sometimes, we are not allowed to use the limb to re-form it, or for someone else. It is wasted. So I sent limbs to Tanzania, for use there.

But now I had more, because people know I try to help others and so they give me their limbs which are finished with. I refuse to throw them away and so I lease a storage unit to store them.

The One Show got to know about Limbcare sending the limbs abroad and contacted us to ask if we were doing the same thing again this year (2013). They asked us where we stored the limbs and were they in a lock-up. This seemed a strange question. I could understand being asked if we were collecting the limbs and sending them elsewhere, but what did it matter to them where we stored them? I asked them why they wanted to know about storage. They told me they were doing a feature about storage units and strange things people store in them. It would seem that a lot of people use lock-ups to store items and they were exploring what was stored in them.

We told them we did have a lock-up and that the limbs were stored in it. Quite strange I suppose, but for us, where else could we store them? The BBC came down to film us in the lock-up with the limbs and did a feature about our collection and distribution of limbs to other countries. We were on *The One Show* showing how we stored the limbs: what we used the lock-up for. I suppose it must be quite surreal really, a whole room full of prosthetic limbs! They filmed me opening the door and all the limbs were there behind me, falling over. The producers were amazed at the wastage, at the fact they could not be used again. I intended to send them to developing countries. I wanted amputees in other countries to have the use of the limbs to help them get on with their lives.

After *The One Show*, for the next five days our support line was so busy, with calls from all over the United Kingdom. Most of the people told us not to send the limbs abroad; there must be a way to keep them. I totally understood the issue, but the health and safety regulations prevented us from using them. It frustrates me too, but I didn't know how to get round it. We then came up with the idea of forming the company Limbcare Recycling. This company strips down the used limbs and the metal parts of the artificial limbs and any items available for scrap will be turned into money that will help fund the Limbcare Apprentice scheme to develop young prosthetists and technicians to follow the experienced people, taking graduates straight from university, training them to produce limbs for the amputee society. It will give us more prosthetists. I realised if I did not do this, the experienced people would retire and we would not have the knowledge passed on. Limbcare can make even better limbs for people. It was so good to meet Matt and Alex. It is ironic, but when I was on the show I met Paul Hollywood, who was advertising his *British Bake-Off*. I remember one conversation when I was showing Matt the artificial limb which is very old, maybe Second World War.

I was given it back and I turned to Paul and said, "Sling that in the oven!"

He just erupted with laughter.

Being on *The One Show* promoted me and Limbcare. I loved it. If it has helped people understand what being disabled is all about then that is why I do what I do.

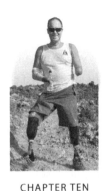

CHAPTER TEN

What next?

Through all the knocks I have had, from the cancer, the septicaemia, the heart attack, everything, people have said to me, "Oh my God, how the hell have you got through it?"

I think it is strength of character and also my dad is in me all the time; it has made me strong and it is a learning curve where I have to be reborn each time. It is like my building blocks are knocked down and then I build them up again, they are knocked down, I build them up again, but I am using reinforcing rods a bit better this time. I am not going to be knocked down so easily any more. All of this gives you a hard shell I and I think it makes you realise life is worth living. I do not suffer fools gladly any more. I can't stand namby-pamby idiots who say they have got colds, who mess about, because that is not in my vocabulary. If you are going to go to work, go to work. I want to work and I do. I think it makes you realise you are among very strong people. When you have had a disability and a knock you learn a big lesson in life. It is a shame, but that makes strength of character.

I think about my mum and how tough things have been for her. She stood by my dad and then watched him die. She has lived through my brother dying and me going through so many illnesses, becoming disabled, and yet she has such strength of character. She says I am one of those people who can cope with everything and I think she is the same. I like sitting with my mum in the garden. She has a lovely little bungalow now in Virginia Water and I do anything for her. It is just great to have my mum around. Let's hope she is here for a long, long time yet.

With regards to my daughters Nicola and Taya, I think basically the icing on the cake appeared through meeting my lovely Fiona, because I was then able to be the dad I wanted to be. However I love all my children and will continue to do so until my dying day. Fiona, bless her, let me be a dad and I know this was more difficult with me having no arms or legs, but I was able to be as independent as I can with the children, and it has been the most enjoyable part of my life, in some ways, so far. There is one extra part which is great: I am now a granddad, thanks to Michael – totally unbelievable and wonderful.

With Nicola and Taya, they have seen me for what I am. When they were babies I used to sit on the sofa, cuddle them and just look at them in awe. Now they are very protective of their daddy. I remember them going to school and their peers saying that their daddy has got plastic arms and taking the mickey a little bit, but the girls gave as good as they got. Now, being someone who is quite high profile in the amputee world, I give talks to schools and I have done that at Nicola and Taya's school. It is good to give back to society what I have gained through a loving marriage and great friendships.

I think if anyone could take a little bit of a leaf out of my book, it's never give up, whatever is thrown in your way. There is always a way of doing things. But I stress, you must communicate. You must talk about it. A problem shared is a problem halved and I was the worst person to talk about things; I bottle them up, and that creates so much frustration and unhappiness. It caused a lot of my problems. If I could turn back time, I would have talked about things more.

You have to have a positive slant on the situation and see the funny side of things. I can remember I was on holiday once and a little boy asked me why I had no arms or legs.

I said to him, "You see this swimming pool you are walking around, early in the morning I dive in and clear all the piranhas and sharks out of the water. One day, unfortunately I got caught."

"You are so brave!"

"That's why the water is so clear!"

"I think you are marvellous!"

He went back to his mum and dad and told them and you can imagine the comments his mum and dad made!

I think that is where children are so fantastic and this is why giving talks to schools in the UK is basically Limbcare education. It is a very proud thing to do. I believe we will go forward, the press is going to follow us, we have been on the BBC's *The One Show,* and my wish is that the publication of this book will raise our profile and make my dream come true.

My story is a blood disorder through poison, but many people suffer amputations through motorbike accidents, car accidents and even food poisoning, leading to septicaemia. But you know it can happen to anybody, we all have to take care. In this modern world we seem to be in a clinical world; everything is so clean! It is not like in the old days when our mums and dads used to go down to the greengrocers and pick up potatoes with a bit of dirt on them. We are not having enough immunity in our system. I think this is where it is causing a lot of problems as well.

I remember the trauma I had when coming from the cotton wool environment of Queen Mary's Hospital Douglas Bader unit to home and you know that story was hell. I had loads of problems. It caused me to get divorced, it caused me to try to commit suicide, it caused me hell on earth. So Limbcare's goal by 2018, with all the help and goodwill of the public, and venture capitalists, is we would like to have a Limbcare Well-Being Centre. This will be a purpose-built building where you can come in, with your family, as a limb-impaired person, feeling lowest of the low, request communication help, just want to talk, want to chill out, want to tell how grief-stricken you are, want help with employment, your limbs not fitting properly, want help with how to go from one place to another, sport, fitness. We will have a lecture theatre for hire where we can also give presentations to professionals to tell them we are there. We want to become part of the rehabilitation team to give people a sense of going forward. This rehabilitation centre will enable people to go in feeling rough and come out saying 'I am pleased it is there'. We may have an accommodation block where a person who has a flat on the third or fourth floor, or whatever, who has had an amputation and cannot go back there because there is no lift, will stay in the accommodation unit until the local authority rehouses them. There is so much to do, but I know this much: if there had been such an organisation when I had my amputations, I know I would have coped with my disability so much better. We need people to understand you can rebuild the body but you cannot rebuild the mind. The whole structure of Limbcare is to get the person to the best quality of life they can get to after a trauma. It will not stop there; Limbcare can grow and grow, but we need your help.

I am so honoured to be the chairman. We now have a new CEO, Dennis, who is one of our trustees. He is an amputee. Barry is still one of our board members. Michael is also a board member and Georgina. All my team are dedicated and I am honoured to be chairman.

All of this needs funding. How do we fund ourselves? Well, the government unfortunately do not help us, but we are lucky enough to have collection days, fund-raising days, e.g. Krispy Kreme days, selling doughnuts, dinner dances, fun fairs and even charities working together to help each other; we are not unique. Why not join forces and help each other to create a togetherness for our charities and what we do? Of course, donating online is important: £5-£50 per month helps us so much, to be able to visit centres and visit amputees to create that new beginning for them. We need officers in every part of the UK. If you are an amputee reading this, please look at the website, please offer your help, because without you we will not be able to help the future amputees of this country. I can only say this: whatever we do, we are a team and whenever you have a united front, you can achieve much more.

I am saying that ambassadors are needed, but you have to have been an amputee for at least 12 months to have coped with your own trauma. If, after then, you feel like giving something back to society, or helping our charity, I would like to speak to you. There are guidelines you have to abide by, because we operate on behalf of a charity and we have to do things right. But as I said before, an amputee helping another amputee is the way forward. I think we owe it to society to help other people. I know we have to live our own lives, but the sense of achievement is more than money can buy, in helping fellow amputees get on with their lives.

On September 27th 2013, we held our Limbcare Gala event. Believe me, it was a team effort and I take my hat off to everyone who helped to organise it and thank them from the bottom of my heart. It is a stepping stone to the future. We launched our Well-Being Centre, which we are trying to raise funds to build in 2018, and there are many places where Limbcare wants to be. I gave the speech of the evening and never realised the mark I would make on the 240 people who were sitting in front of me. You could hear a pin drop during my speech and I could have had everyone eating out of my hand. I felt very honoured and proud to say the words I did and it came from the heart. I believe this is the transition from where Ray was to where Ray is going. The room was buzzing, there was so much interest and I do not think our guests realised what Limbcare was about until I spoke. It was very emotional for all.

From my point of view, I am lucky that I am a fairly good communicator and I give motivational and inspirational speeches. I have had the honour of giving talks in parliament, to high profile companies and to schools and, believe me, meeting young people from the age of four up to 18 is wonderful because they are our future and children are our greatest ambassadors. They ask questions, you give the right answer and they go away.

As with any business, be it a charity or whatever, you are going to get trials and tribulations. Getting finance for a start, how to deal with people. You never please everybody, there is a saying: 'You can please some people some of the time, but you can't please all the people all of the time'. I try to please everybody and over the years I should have learned by now that it is a bloody impossible way to do things. As I am now the chairman, I look at the team and think *Well, they have to make mistakes to learn and they have to understand that we all travel in different ways but as long as we all know we are singing from the same hymn sheet, we as a team will create something unique.* And I don't think there is any other organisation, charity, whatever, with a quad amputee who has gone through so much at the helm and with as many passionate people as we have in our team. It is just a unique and beautiful, beautiful organisation.

When you come to dealing with problems, you have to rise above them. Everybody has good qualities and I know through my own experiences that sometimes there is a lot of insecurity in the world. People do not know how to communicate. The best communicators I have met are wheelchair-bound people. I think disability is in the eye of the beholder, and in this 21st century we are all the same – amputees, people with disability of any kind – and it is a unique opportunity to be able to work together. We must not segregate and pigeonhole people. We, as Limbcare, advocate a united front on this. I hope to God that one day we will have a big voice in the government to help everybody in the prosthetic industry in the UK, to provide the quality of life people should expect when they become an amputee.

Since all my trauma and really hitting rock bottom and coming out of the gloom, I believe that I am special and I have been guided to do things to help people of all ages. I am particularly focused on young people. I like to visit schools to give the children an insight into what disability is all about. I am very fortunate in being able to communicate well and describe certain traumas in a way children can understand and relate to.

In my position now, as chairman of Limbcare, it has dawned on me that we can help children through my speaking as well through the charity. From this, we have formed Limbcare Youth.

Life has dealt me some terrible cards and I played the game the best I could, but the question is now, where is Ray? What is Ray? Who is Ray? He is a man who is destined now to help others, to give inspiration and hope. Funnily enough, I didn't realise how powerful I am in regards to people taking away an inspirational thought: that Ray has got everywhere through adversity and traumas of life and he is giving hope to everyone he meets. In particular, I meet people who go away feeling much better in themselves. What a gift! I never realised I had that. But what am I going to do in the future? Well, I love Limbcare, but that is not the end, it is the beginning. I see myself as an inspirational and motivational speaker, especially giving talks to children which I love to do all the time.

In the last couple of months I have had many, many enquiries requesting me to visit schools, to talk to the children who are, of course, our ambassadors. They take away everything and don't ask questions and when they do, they ask them and that is it. In other words, they see me as a quad amputee, they ask questions of where and how it all happened and then they take it on board and that is it. The trouble is as adults we don't question. We look and then we go into our own shell, thinking *I must not ask*. I think that is wrong because society as a whole needs to communicate much better, to become an informative world. Through the education part of my life, giving talks and presentations, it is helping me. I must say I feel better with my life when I am talking to others about themselves. I wish I could look after myself at times, because I don't. I do not look after what Ray really wants. I do take a back seat on things now, thinking I have to be happy, because if I am happy, the world is happy.

I'd love this book to inspire people as to how the world deals with amputees and disabled people. No one wants to be reclusive. We all want to be loved. The way I look at it I am open, I am truthful and I am forthright in a way and I certainly don't care for people who whinge. Life has brought this on me and I am making the best of my disability. I don't feel I am disabled; I feel I have been sent a lifeline which has been traumatic, but has made me an inspirational leader to help others. My flock, like a shepherd's, is increasing all the time. I am very, very proud to be alive and I believe my destiny is to travel around the UK and maybe the world, giving talks and conferences, after-dinner speaking, really telling people what it is all about. That is one thing I am good at, talking to people.

In between all the positive days, there are bound to be negative ones – it is the same for everyone. We all think a lot, our memory bank is so clever and do I ever think, or wish, things were different? Of course I do! But when I have time to reflect on what I have got, I seriously think now I wouldn't change very much. I have beautiful children, a lovely wife, friends, and I think the journey I have been on is quite unique.

One thing I have to do is juggle my life to be with my family, because without Fiona and my children, life wouldn't be the same. Now is the time to have a bit of 'me' time. It is nice to chill out. I like to swim, which I can do in the summer, but in the winter I walk. It is good when you are walking, meeting people, because it dawns on people that even with artificial limbs, especially legs, you can still get on with life. This is my new life and Ray is going to make it a happier place!

I think Limbcare has been the diving board, the key to my new world. Limbcare was meant to be, to create my new world.

If I had stayed as the old Ray Edwards, yes I would have been a very rich, successful builder, a pain in the arse, but not devoted to helping others. I would not be on this new journey to create a better life for amputees. I do think, in a way, that these battles I fought were all meant to be and have truly made me what I am today.

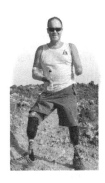

What others say!

What can I say about the care and support I have received from Limbcare during a recent time of great trial?

Due to a chronic condition caused by radiotherapy I received way back in 1976, my right lower leg had always been a problem, with amputation an ever present option. Come 2005 a successful flap surgery saved my limb again. However, over the course of 2013 the situation deteriorated rapidly following an unsuccessful attempt by my skilled plastic surgeons to repair an enormous ulcer on my shin and spreading necrosis through my foot.

I was then faced with the terrifying prospect of losing the limb and was sent home by the surgical team to make the decision to carry on as I was – hobbling on sticks, enduring ever increasing pain, a lifetime of painkilling drugs and antibiotics, stinky dressings to be changed four times a week at my local doctor's and the ever present threat of infection or even the potentially lethal septicaemia – OR take the plunge and face the scenario I feared most since 1976: 'a shortening of the limb' – the innocuous term for amputation!

On the face of it, an easy decision but one that, no matter how obvious, had petrified me from the outset of my difficulties in 1976.

Enter stage right – from Limbcare the Mighty Mighty – the force of nature that is known as Ray Edwards MBE (no less).

Ray arrived and took me for coffee. What an inspiration! friendly, empathetic chat ensued where my fears were calmed and qualms dissipated. He was certainly rocking the look with all prostheses clearly on show and drawing admiring looks and comments from the staff and customers at Go-Gos, Dedworth Road, Windsor (best coffee and bacon butties for miles).

Why should I be in such a dark place anticipating just one small amputation when there was a clear example of how someone not only survives such an operation but actually thrives and achieves? But there I was, lacking the confidence to give the go-ahead for my potentially life-enhancing operation.

Ray then arranged for the Mighty Mighty Dennis Outridge to do a home visit. Dennis had been in exactly the same position as me: self-elected amputation right leg below knee.

Here was a man not averse to dropping his trousers to show the logistics of prosthesis and showing off his star jumps to demonstrate his agility. I sat nearby unable to stagger more than a few feet on agonized toes, more disabled than he could ever be!

Fast forward to August 2013 and with my operation complete after the agonizing decision was made. Sat in the day room of Ward 2 Wexham Park Hospital, both Ray and Dennis have taken time out to visit me. This is their last stop before home following a full business day up north. I am presented with my badge of honour – my Limbcare bracelet.

It's a good club to be in. Rather that than the Agonising Pain, Smelly Dressing, Completely Incapacitated club I was previously a card-carrying member of and reluctant to give up that membership!

Limbcare offered support, information, advice and above all inspiration. I strongly viewed my situation as THE END. Limbcare, by personal example, showed it merely as transition – another fulfilling life awaits.

Thank you Limbcare, Ray and Dennis. You are definitely at the very top of my Windsor August 2013 Whatabloke list, beating the likes of Mott the Hoople, Sherlock Holmes, Batman and Doctor Who.

You were with me when a vital decision was required and there at the aftermath when further support was appreciated.

Thank you from the bottom of my heart.

Julian Turner Bell

Help for Heros.

We have learned much from Ray Edwards MBE and his experience of being a quad amputee. I hope that H4H and Limbcare can work closely together to share and learn how to rise above adversity.

Bryn Parry - *Founder H4H*

Glenesk School

In June this year Ray Edwards came to school to talk to the children about his life as a quad amputee. They watched with fascination as he explained how he had overcome illness as a teenager and after contracting septicaemia learnt to walk again with the use of artificial limbs. The children followed Ray along his trek up Kilimanjaro and his determination to conquer something which would normally be beyond the reach of many!

Ray's talk not only motivated the children to arrange a triathlon to raise money for Limbcare, but also left them with a greater understanding and empathy for others.

Ray is truly inspirational and taught the children the most valuable lesson that anything is possible if you believe in yourself and never give up. He gained many friends that day and memories of him running and cycling with the children will remain with them for ever!

Glenesk School
Surrey 2012

Cardiff 2011

I was invited to give a presentation to third year occupational therapy students at Cardiff and was delighted to accept. I have always felt that education is so important and to let these young people see and understand what life is like to live as a quad amputee is paramount in their approach to becoming an OT. I was honoured to do this and afterwards questions were flying, the room buzzed. This was a great feeling. Ruth Squire, the lecturer, thanked me and was very proud and inspired by my presence and presentation. She hopes I can return again.

Naidex

I have always attended Naidex every year in Birmingham to witness the latest technology for making life easier for disabled and carers. This year I was asked by the organisers to give a presentation. Of course I accepted with pleasure. Again the presentation that I gave was inspirational and went down well with many attendees of the Naidex, able bodied and disabled including wheelchair users. I was elated with the applause and very interesting questions were asked

"Ray spoke to my sales team at a recent get-together. I found the him to be inspirational and motivational whilst retaining a sense of humour"

Chris Maylon DSV

*I found the Limbcare presentation informative
and inspirational.*

– Natasha Balloch

*I found the Limbcare talk very refreshing to see a
charity wishing to provide both the practical and
emotional support to not only the physical sufferer
but also to family and friends.*

– Steph Langdon-Goff

*The Limbcare presentation was excellent and very
informative. I would not hesitate to provide clients
with their details in the future.*

– Abbie Hickson

*I feel honoured to have had the opportunity to meet
Ray Edwards and his team to listen to their stories.
Ray made me want to cry and laugh at the same
time. His story is amazing and he is inspirational.
He gave me a real insight into the immense
difficulties faced by amputees, but also the amazing
things they can and do achieve (trust me when I say
I could never climb Mount Kilimanjaro!).
I think everyone would benefit from taking the time
to hear this talk.*

– Gilly Jones

Most interesting – Limbcare presentation.

– Rachel Seddon

I really enjoyed hearing about Limbcare.
Ray and his colleagues are a breath of fresh air!

– Sarah Lake

Limbcare is a worthwhile and notable cause.

– Simon Dueck

Limbcare were really informative. I really enjoyed
their talk and would feel confident in referring
a client for help.

– Morag Lewis

Ray and his team at Limbcare were informative
and inspirational. Their mixture of humour and
real life examples really got the message across that
we need to do more for those affected by limb loss.

– Debra Woolfson

Limbcare – very inspirational talk.

– Shelley Nedimovic

A final THANK YOU to the Sponsors of this book, who
have made the publishing of it possible:

Sue Christie Hall and Friends of Glenesk School

Maureen Brosnahan

Cherryl and Richard Little

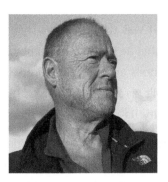

About the author

Ray Edwards MBE was born in 1954 near London. He had a relatively ordinary life: the eldest son of a builder, he followed his father to work for the family company and thought life was good until at 27 years old he found out he had cancer. He had treatment, including an operation, chemotherapy and radiotherapy, which was successful, the only downfall being he could not father children, or so he was told. This was proved to be untrue, as Ray then went on to father twins, much to the delight of both Ray and his wife.

It was while back at work, when the twins were under a year old, that Ray cut his hand. Within 24 hours life had changed for Ray, who developed septicaemia. To save his life, both arms and both legs had to be amputated. He was also on a kidney dialysis machine.

Ray went through many lows in his struggle to get back to be the person he was, including the breakdown of his first marriage. It was while he was trying to get his life back together that he had a vision of helping others in his position: amputees and limb impaired. He also married someone he calls his angel who helped him come to term with his disability. Ray also has three more children.

Ray has worked with several charities in pursuit of helping amputees and was awarded the MBE for his services. He is now the chairman of Limbcare, a charity supporting amputees and limb impaired of all ages. He is also an inspirational speaker, travelling the country inspiring everyone.

This book was written not only to give people inspiration, whatever their circumstances, to get the most out of life, but also to support Limbcare.

Ray is already beginning to write his second book about the journey Limbcare is on and his recent adventures in the promotion of Limbcare, including his appearance on television.

For more information:
www.ray-inspires.org
www.limbcare.org

Lightning Source UK Ltd.
Milton Keynes UK
UKOW07f0017221114

242013UK00001B/2/P